HANDBOOK OF
NURSING DIAGNOSIS
1989–90

Handbook of Nursing Diagnosis 1989–90

Lynda Juall Carpenito, R.N., M.S.N.

Nursing Consultant, Mickleton, New Jersey

J. B. Lippincott Company   Philadelphia

Cambridge New York St Louis San Francisco

London Singapore Sydney Tokyo

Acquisition/Sponsoring Editor: Nancy Mullins
Coordinating Editorial Assistant: Ellen Campbell
Manuscript Editor: Lee Henderson
Indexer: Ellen Murray
Design Coordinator: Michelle Gerdes
Cover Designer: Wendy Cummiskey
Production Manager: Carol A. Florence
Production Coordinator: Kathryn Rule
Compositor: TAPSCO, Inc.
Printer/Binder: R. R. Donnelley & Sons Company
Cover Printer: New England Book Components

3 5 6 4 2

Library of Congress Cataloging-in-Publication Data

Carpenito, Lynda Juall.
    Handbook of nursing diagnosis, 1989–90/Lynda Juall Carpenito.
        p.   cm.
    Includes index.
    ISBN 0-397-54763-3
    1. Diagnosis—Handbooks, manuals, etc.   2. Nursing—Hand-
books, manuals, etc.   I. Title.
    [DNLM: 1. Nursing Assessment—handbooks.   WY 39 C294h]
RT48.C365 1989   88-23089
616.075—dc19   CIP

To Olen, my son

for your innocence and wisdom
for our quiet moments and sudden hugs
for your unsolicited distractions
. . . I am grateful

for you are my daily reminder of what is
really important . . .
love, health, and human trust

Acknowledgments

I would like to thank the following people for their consultation during the development of the manual:

Rosalinda Alfaro, R.N., M.S.N.
Lecturer
Immaculata College
Immaculata, Pennsylvania;
Per Diem Staff Nurse
Intensive Care Units
Paoli Memorial Hospital
Paoli, Pennsylvania

Cynthia Balin, R.N., M.S.N.
Director of Clinical Services
Kissimmee Memorial Hospital
Kissimmee, Florida

Martha Cress, R.N., B.S.N.
Nursing Education and Development
Duke University Medical Center
Durham, North Carolina

Ann Curtis, R.N., B.S.N.
Staff Development Department
Wilmington Medical Center
Wilmington, Delaware

Jacqueline W. Levett, R.N., M.S.N.
Pediatric Clinical Specialist
Wilmington Medical Center
Wilmington, Delaware

Mary Sieggreen, R.N., M.S.N., C.S.
Case Manager
Surgical Product Line
Harper Hospital
Detroit, Michigan

Mary Mishler Vogel, R.N., M.S.N.
Instructor
Helene Fuld School of Nursing
Camden, New Jersey

Joan Wagger, R.N., M.S.N.
Nursing Education and Development
Duke University Medical Center
Durham, North Carolina

Anne E. Willard, R.N., M.S.N.
Associate Professor
Cumberland County College
Vineland, New Jersey

A sincere "thank you" to my diligent typist,
Maria Manel; to Lee Henderson for his precise
editing; and once again, to my husband,
Richard, for his support on yet another project.

Acknowledgments

Contents

Contents

x

Contents

Section II
DIAGNOSTIC CLUSTERS
(Medical Diagnostic Categories
With Associated Nursing Diagnoses
and Collaborative Problems)

Total Parenteral Nutrition (Hyperalimentation)

Contents

Psychiatric Disorders 322

Introduction

DIAGNOSTIC CATEGORIES

In 1973, the North American Nursing Diagnosis Association (NANDA; formerly, the National Group for the Classification of Nursing Diagnosis) published its first list of nursing diagnoses. Since that time, the interest in nursing diagnosis and its application in clinical settings has grown substantially. In the 1970s, the main issue in nursing centered on the value of establishing a classification system for nursing diagnoses. Now that there is general agreement about the need for a formal taxonomy, the current issue is the implementation of nursing diagnoses. The challenge that nurses face today is one of identifying specific nursing diagnoses for those people assigned to their care and of incorporating these diagnoses into a plan of care.

This handbook does not focus on teaching nurses about the concept of nursing diagnosis. For information describing the concept and specific instructions for clinical use the reader is referred to Carpenito LJ: Nursing Diagnosis: Application to Clinical Practice, 3rd ed. Philadelphia, JB Lippincott, 1989.

This handbook is intended to supplement texts on nursing diagnosis in two ways:

- By providing a quick reference to each diagnostic category in terms of its definition, defining characteristics, and etiological, contributing, and risk factors
- By identifying possible nursing diagnoses and collaborative problems that could be associated with the major medical diagnoses

Section I consists of 100 diagnostic categories, including 88 approved by NANDA and 12 additional categories. The additional categories are

Altered Bowel Elimination
Total Self-care Deficit
Altered Comfort
Pruritis
Nausea/Vomiting
Self-concept Disturbance
Grieving

Impaired Communication
Potential for Infection Transmission
Potential Altered Respiratory Function
Potential for Self-harm
Maturational Enuresis

Each diagnostic category is described in terms of

- Definition
- Defining characteristics, which are the clinical
  criteria that represent the presence of the diagnosis (actual or potential). Defining characteristics for actual nursing diagnoses are a single
  sign or symptom or a cluster of signs and symptoms. Categories with clinical validation studies
  have major signs and symptoms present 80%
  of the time, minor signs and symptoms 50% to
  79% of the time. The *major* category includes
  those signs and symptoms that must be present
  to validate use of a diagnosis. The *minor* classification refers to characteristics that appear to
  be present in many but not all individuals experiencing the diagnosis. Minor characteristics
  are not less serious than the major ones; they
  are just not present in all individuals. For potential nursing diagnoses the defining characteristics are the presence of risk factors.
- Etiological, contributing, and risk factors, which
  are examples of pathophysiological, treatment-
  related, situational, and maturational factors
  that can cause or influence the health status or
  contribute to the development of a problem

ACTUAL, POTENTIAL, AND POSSIBLE NURSING DIAGNOSES

A nursing diagnosis can be actual, potential, or possible.

Actual: An actual nursing diagnosis describes a
diagnostic category that the nurse has
validated because of the presence of major
defining characteristics, or signs and
symptoms.

Potential: A potential nursing diagnosis
describes an altered state that may occur if

certain nursing interventions are not
ordered and implemented.

Possible: A possible nursing diagnosis describes
a problem that the nurse suspects may be
present but that requires additional data
collection to confirm or rule out its
presence.

DIAGNOSTIC STATEMENTS

The diagnostic statement describes the health status
of an individual or group and the factors that have
contributed to the status.

Statement of health status		Factors that have contributed
↓		↓
Diagnostic category	Related to	Contributing/ risk factors
↓	↓	↓
Fear	Related to	Unknown prognosis secondary to cancer diagnosis

The diagnostic statement or the nursing diagnosis
should consist of two or three parts.

Two-part Statements

Potential and possible nursing diagnoses have two
parts. The validation for a potential nursing diagnosis
is the presence of risk factors. The risk factors are the
second part.

Potential nursing diagnosis   Related to   Risk factors

Possible nursing diagnoses are suspected because
of the presence of certain factors. The nurse then
either rules out or confirms the existence of an actual
or a potential diagnosis.

Examples of two-part statements are

Potential Impairment of Skin Integrity related to
immobility secondary to fractured hip
Possible Self-care Deficit related to impaired
ability to use left hand secondary to IV

Designating a diagnosis as possible provides the nurse with a method to communicate to other nurses that a diagnosis may be present. Additional data collection is indicated to rule out or confirm the tentative diagnosis.

Three-part Statements

An actual nursing diagnosis consists of three parts.

> Diagnostic label + contributing factors + signs and symptoms

The presence of major signs and symptoms (defining characteristics) validates that an actual diagnosis is present. It is not possible to have a third part for potential or possible diagnoses because signs and symptoms do not exist.

Examples of three-part statements are

Anxiety related to unpredictable nature of asthmatic episodes as manifested by statements of "I'm afraid I won't be able to breathe"

Urge Incontinence related to diminished bladder capacity secondary to habitual frequent voiding as manifested by inability to hold off urination after desire to void and report of voiding out of habit, not need

The presence of a nursing diagnosis is determined by assessing the individual's health status and his ability to function. To guide the nurse who is gathering this information, a Data-base Assessment Tool is included in the Appendix at the end of the book. This guide directs the nurse to collect data according to the individual's functional health patterns. Functional health patterns and the corresponding nursing diagnoses are listed in Table 2, at the end of this introduction. If significant data are collected in a particular functional pattern, the next step is to check the related diagnostic categories to see if any nursing diagnoses are substantiated by the data that are collected.

Section II of this handbook consists of seven parts: (1) Medical Diagnoses, (2) Surgical Procedures, (3) Obstetrical/Gynecological Conditions, (4) Neonatal

Conditions, (5) Pediatric/Adolescent Disorders, (6) Psychiatric Disorders, and (7) Diagnostic and Therapeutic Procedures. Each of these subjects is represented by a series of diagnostic categories under which groups of associated nursing diagnoses and collaborative problems are listed. The intent of this section is to help the nurse identify possible nursing diagnoses in each of these areas. It is important to note that each nursing diagnosis must be confirmed or ruled out on the basis of the data collected. The use of a nursing diagnosis without clinical validation based on defining characteristics is hazardous and unsound, and jeopardizes the effectiveness and validity of the nursing care plan. The listing of tentative nursing diagnoses under medical and surgical diagnoses was intended to facilitate the assessment, identification, and validation process, *not to replace it.*

In addition to the possible nursing diagnoses listed under each medical category, there is a list of potential collaborative problems or complications that may occur.

Nursing interventions address two types of problems—those described by nursing diagnoses and collaborative problems.

A *nursing diagnosis* is a statement that describes the human response of an individual or group to life processes so that the nurse can legally identify the response and can then order the definitive interventions to promote the health state or to reduce, eliminate, or prevent alterations from health.

Collaborative problems are physiological complications for which nurses use monitoring skills to detect onset or status so that nursing can collaborate with medicine to provide definitive co-treatment.

The nurse makes independent decisions regarding both collaborative problems and nursing diagnoses. The decisions differ in that, for nursing diagnoses, the nurse prescribes most of the definitive treatment for the situation; for collaborative problems the nurse primarily monitors the patient's condition to detect onset or status of physiological complications to prevent a worsened condition or death. When a nurse diagnoses a collaborative problem, the nurse confers with the physician regarding treatment. When a nurse makes a nursing diagnosis, this collaboration is usually not warranted. Rather than make up new titles for interdependent situations, collaborative problems can simply be labeled "Potential Complication:" (specify).

Examples:

Potential Complication: Hemorrhage
Potential Complication: Renal Failure

The physiological complications that nurses monitor are usually related to disease, trauma, treatments, and diagnostic studies. The following illustrates some collaborative problems for which monitoring is needed (if the situation warrants monitoring for detection of a cluster or group of physiological complications, the problem can be documented as "Potential Complication: Cardiac"):

Situation	Collaborative Problem
Anticoagulant therapy	Potential Complication: Hemorrhage
NPO state	Potential Complication: Hypovolemia/hypervolemia
Pneumonia	Potential Complication: Hypoxia

Table 1 is a list of frequently used collaborative problems.

Some physiological complications, such as pressure ulcers and infection from invasive lines, are problems that nurses can prevent. Prevention is different from detection. Nurses do not prevent paralytic ileus but, instead, detect its presence early to prevent greater severity of illness or even death. Physicians cannot treat collaborative problems without nursing knowledge, vigilance, and judgment. In situations requiring prevention, nurses institute orders in addition to monitoring, such as ordering position changes, patient teaching, or specific protocols.

Thus the type of intervention differentiates a nursing diagnosis from a collaborative problem and also differentiates an actual nursing diagnosis from a po-

Table 1. Frequently Used Collaborative Problems

1. **Potential Complication: Gastrointestinal/Hepatic**

   Potential Complication: Paralytic Ileus/Small Bowel Obstruction

   Potential Complication: Hepatorenal Syndrome

   Potential Complication: Hyperbilirubenia

   Potential Complication: Evisceration

   Potential Complication: Hepatosplenomegaly

   Potential Complication: Curling's Ulcer

   Potential Complication: Ascites

   Potential Complication: Gastrointestinal Bleeding

2. **Potential Complication: Metabolic/Immune**

   Potential Complication: Hypoglycemia

   Potential Complication: Hyperglycemia

   Potential Complication: Negative Nitrogen Balance

   Potential Complication: Electrolyte Imbalances

   Potential Complication: Thyroid Dysfunction

   Potential Complication: Hypoglycemia (Severe)

   Potential Complication: Hyperthermia (Severe)

   Potential Complication: Sepsis

   Potential Complication: Acidosis/Alkalosis

   Potential Complication: Diabetes

   Potential Complication: Anasarca

   Potential Complication: Hypothyroidism/Hyperthyroidism

   Potential Complication: Allergic Reaction

   Potential Complication: Donor Tissue Rejection

   Potential Complication: Adrenal Insufficiency

3. **Potential Complication: Neurological/Sensory**

   Potential Complication: Increased Intracranial Pressure

   Potential Complication: Stroke

   Potential Complication: Seizures

   Potential Complication: Spinal Cord Compression

   Potential Complication: Autonomic Dysreflexia

   Potential Complication: Birth Injuries

   Potential Complication: Hydrocephalus

   Potential Complication: Microcephalus

   Potential Complication: Meningitis

   Potential Complication: Cranial Nerve Impairment

   Potential Complication: Paresis/Paresthesia/Paralysis

   (Continued)

Table 1. Frequently Used Collaborative Problems (*Continued*)

Potential Complication: Peripheral Nerve Impairment

Potential Complication: Increased Intraocular Pressure

Potential Complication: Corneal Ulceration

Potential Complication: Neuropathies

4. Potential Complication: Cardiovascular

Potential Complication: Dysrhythmias

Potential Complication: Congestive Heart Failure

Potential Complication: Cardiogenic Shock

Potential Complication: Thromboemboli/Deep Vein Thrombosis

Potential Complication: Hypovolemic Shock

Potential Complication: Peripheral Vascular Insufficiency

Potential Complication: Hypertension

Potential Complication: Congenital Heart Disease

Potential Complication: Thrombocytopenia

Potential Complication: Polycythemia

Potential Complication: Anemia

Potential Complication: Compartmental Syndrome

Potential Complication: Disseminated Intravascular Coagulation

Potential Complication: Endocarditis

Potential Complication: Sickling Crisis

Potential Complication: Embolism (air, fat)

Potential Complication: Spinal Shock

Potential Complication: Ischemic Ulcers

5. Potential Complication: Respiratory

Potential Complication: Atelectasis/Pneumonia

Potential Complication: Asthma

Potential Complication: Chronic Obstructive Pulmonary Disease

Potential Complication: Pulmonary Embolism

Potential Complication: Pleural Effusion

Potential Complication: Tracheal Necrosis

Potential Complication: Ventilator Dependency

Potential Complication: Pneumothorax

Potential Complication: Laryngeal Edema

Potential Complication: Pneumothorax

6. Potential Complication: Renal/Urinary

Potential Complication: Acute Urinary Retention

(Continued)

Table 1. Frequently Used Collaborative Problems *(Continued)*

Potential Complication:	Renal Failure
Potential Complication:	Bladder Perforation
7. Potential Complication:	**Reproductive**
Potential Complication:	Fetal Compromise
Potential Complication:	Uterine Atony
Potential Complication:	Pregnancy-induced Hypertension
Potential Complication:	Eclampsia
Potential Complication:	Hydraminos
Potential Complication:	Hypermenorrhea
Potential Complication:	Polymenorrhea
Potential Complication:	Syphilis
8. Potential Complication:	**Musculoskeletal**
Potential Complication:	Stress Fractures
Potential Complication:	Osteoporosis
Potential Complication:	Joint Dislocation

tential or possible one. Below are definitions of each type and the corresponding intervention focus:

Type	Focus of Nursing Interventions
Actual (is present)	To reduce, eliminate, or promote (positive) and monitor
Potential (may happen)	To prevent onset and monitor
Possible (may be present)	To rule out or confirm with additional data
Collaborative Problem	To monitor onset or status

For example, for the diagnosis Impaired Skin Integrity related to immobility as manifested by a 2-cm epidermal lesion on the left heel, the nurse would order interventions to monitor the lesion while providing care to eliminate it. Monitoring is an intervention used for all diagnoses. If the outcome criteria for a problem necessitate medical interventions and the nursing focus is primarily on monitoring or surveillance, perhaps a nursing diagnosis is inappropriate because a collaborative problem is present. Nursing diagnoses are not more important than collaborative problems, and collaborative problems are not more important than nursing diagnoses. Rather, priorities are determined by the client's situation.

How to Use the Manual

1. Collect data, both subjective and objective, from client, family, other health care professionals, and records. (Refer to Appendix: Adult Database Assessment Guide.)
2. Identify a possible pattern or problem.
3. Refer to the medical diagnostic category and review the possible associated nursing diagnoses and collaborative problems. Select the possibilities.
4. After you have selected what physiological complications or collaborative problems are indicated to be monitored for, label them Potential Complications: (specify).
5. After you have determined which functional patterns are altered or at risk of altered functioning, review the list of nursing diagnostic categories under that pattern and select the appropriate diagnosis (refer to Table 2).
6. If you select an actual diagnosis,
   - Do you have signs and symptoms to support its presence? (Refer to Section I, Nursing Diagnostic Categories, under the selected diagnosis.)
   - Write the actual diagnosis in three parts: Category related to contributing factors as manifested by signs and symptoms
7. If you select a potential diagnosis
   - Are risk factors present?
   - Write the potential diagnosis in two parts: Category related to risk factors
8. If you suspect a problem but have insufficient data, gather the additional data to confirm or rule out the diagnosis. If this additional data collection must be done later or by other nurses, label the diagnosis *possible* on the care plan.*

* Specific focus assessment criteria questions, outcome criteria, and interventions for each nursing diagnosis category can be found in Carpenito LJ: Nursing Diagnosis: Application to Clinical Practice, 3rd ed. Philadelphia, JB Lippincott, 1989.

Table 2. Nursing Diagnostic Categories Grouped Under Functional Health Patterns*

1. **Health Perception–Health Management**
   †Breastfeeding, Ineffective
   Growth and Development, Altered
   Health Maintenance, Altered
   †Health Seeking Behaviors
   Noncompliance
   Potential for Injury
      Potential for Suffocation
      Potential for Poisoning
      Potential for Trauma

2. **Nutritional–Metabolic**
   Body Temperature, Potential Altered
      Hypothermia
      Hyperthermia
      Thermoregulation, Ineffective
   Fluid Volume Deficit
   Fluid Volume Excess
   Infection, Potential for
   ‡Infection Transmission, Potential for
   Nutrition, Altered: Less Than Body
      Requirements
   Nutrition, Altered: More Than Body
      Requirements
   Nutrition, Altered: Potential for More Than Body
      Requirements
      Swallowing, Impaired
   Tissue Integrity, Impaired
      Oral Mucous Membrane, Altered
      Skin Integrity, Impaired

3. **Elimination**
   ‡Bowel Elimination, Altered
      Constipation
      †Colonic Constipation
      †Perceived Constipation
      Diarrhea
      Bowel Incontinence
   Urinary Elimination, Altered Patterns of
      Urinary Retention
      Total Incontinence

(Continued)

Table 2. Nursing Diagnostic Categories Grouped Under Functional Health Patterns (Continued)

Functional Incontinence
Reflex Incontinence
Urge Incontinence
Stress Incontinence
‡Maturational Enuresis

4. **Activity–Exercise**
   Activity Intolerance
   Cardiac Output, Decreased
   †Disuse Syndrome, Potential for
   Diversional Activity Deficit
   Home Maintenance Management, Impaired
   Mobility, Impaired Physical
   ‡Respiratory Function, Potential Altered
      Ineffective Airway Clearance
      Ineffective Breathing Patterns
      Impaired Gas Exchange
   (Specify) Self-care Deficit: (Total,‡ Feeding,
      Bathing/Hygiene, Dressing/Grooming,
      Toileting)
   Tissue Perfusion, Altered: (Specify) (Cerebral,
      Cardiopulmonary, Renal, Gastrointestinal,
      Peripheral)

5. **Sleep–Rest**
   Sleep Pattern Disturbance

6. **Cognitive–Perceptual**
   ‡Comfort, Altered
      Pain
      ‡Acute Pain
      Chronic Pain
      ‡Pruritus
      ‡Nausea/Vomiting
   †Decisional Conflict
   †Dysreflexia
   Knowledge Deficit: (Specify)
   †Potential for Aspiration
   Sensory–Perceptual Alteration: (Specify) (Visual,
      Auditory, Kinesthetic, Gustatory, Tactile,
      Olfactory)

(Continued)

Thought Processes, Altered
Unilateral Neglect

7. **Self-Perception**
   Anxiety
   †Fatigue
   Fear
   Hopelessness
   Powerlessness
   ‡Self-concept Disturbance
      Body Image Disturbance
      Personal Identity Disturbance
      †Self-esteem Disturbance
         †Chronic Low Self-esteem
         †Situational Low Self-esteem

8. **Role–Relationship**
   ‡Communication, Impaired
      Communication, Impaired Verbal
   Family Processes, Altered
   ‡Grieving
      Grieving, Anticipatory
      Grieving, Dysfunctional
   Parenting, Altered
   †Parental Role Conflict
   Role Performance, Altered
   Social Interactions, Impaired
   Social Isolation

9. **Sexuality–Reproductive**
   Sexual Dysfunction
   Sexuality Patterns, Altered

10. **Coping–Stress Tolerance**
    Adjustment, Impaired
    Coping, Ineffective Individual
       †Defensive Coping
       †Ineffective Denial
    Coping: Disabling, Ineffective Family
    Coping: Compromised, Ineffective Family
    Coping: Potential for Growth, Family

(*Continued*)

Table 2. Nursing Diagnostic Categories Grouped Under Functional Health Patterns* (Continued)

Post-trauma Response
Rape Trauma Syndrome
‡Self-harm, Potential for:
Violence, Potential for:

11. Value–Belief
Spiritual Distress

---

*The Functional Health Patterns were identified in Gordon M: Nursing Diagnosis: Process and Application. New York, McGraw-Hill, 1982, with minor changes by the author.
†These categories were accepted by the North American Nursing Diagnosis Association in 1988.
‡These diagnostic categories are not currently on the NANDA list but have been included for clarity and usefulness.

HANDBOOK OF
NURSING DIAGNOSIS
1989-90

Section I

Nursing Diagnostic Categories

Activity Intolerance

DEFINITION

Activity Intolerance: The state in which the individual experiences an inability, physiologically and psychologically, to endure or tolerate an increase in activity.

DEFINING CHARACTERISTICS

Major (Must Be Present)

Altered response to activity
  Respiratory
    Dyspnea
    Shortness of
        breath
  Pulse
    Weak
    Decrease in rate
    Excessive increase
        in rate

  Blood pressure
    Failure to
        increase with
        activity
    Increase in
        diastolic by
        15 mm Hg
  Weakness
  Fatigue

Excessive increase
    in rate
Decrease in rate

Failure to return
    to resting
    after three
    minutes
Rhythm change

Decrease

Minor (May Be Present)

  Pallor or cyanosis
  Confusion
  Vertigo

ETIOLOGICAL, CONTRIBUTING, RISK FACTORS

Any factor that compromises oxygen transport can cause activity intolerance. Some common factors are listed below.

Pathophysiological

Alterations in the oxygen transport system
  Cardiac
    Congestive heart failure   Angina
    Arrhythmias   Myocardial infarction
  Respiratory
    Chronic obstructive pulmonary disease
  Circulatory
    Anemia
    Peripheral arterial disease
  Acute infection
    Viral infection
    Mononucleosis
    Hepatitis
  Chronic infection
    Endocarditis
    Tuberculosis
  Endocrine or metabolic disorders
    Diabetes mellitus
    Hypothyroidism
    Pituitary disorders
    Addison's disease
  Chronic diseases
    Renal   Inflammatory
    Hepatic   Musculoskeletal
         Neurological

  Nutritional disorders
    Obesity
    Malnourishment
    Inadequate diet
  Hypovolemia
  Electrolyte imbalance
  Malignancies

Treatment-related

Surgery
Diagnostic studies
Treatment schedule/treatments (frequency)
Prolonged bed rest
Medications
  Antihypertensives
  Minor tranquilizers
  Hypnotics
  Antidepressants
  Antihistamines

Situational (Personal, Environmental)

Depression
Lack of motivation
Sedentary life-style
Extreme stress
Crisis—personal or developmental, career,
    family, financial
Stressors (*e.g.*)

Impaired language function	Impaired motor function
Impaired sensory function	Pain

Fatigue
Caused by (*e.g.*)

Sensory overload	Equipment that requires strength (walkers, crutches, braces)
Sensory deprivation	
Interrupted sleep	
	Stress

Maturational

Elderly (sensory-motor deficit)

Adjustment, Impaired

DEFINITION

Impaired Adjustment: The state in which an individual is unable to modify his/her life-style/behavior in a manner consistent with a change in health status.

> **Author's Note:**
>
> The term *adjustment* describes an individual's psychosocial regulatory processes to establish equilibrium in a person-environment. This individual is having difficulty adapting to a health status change.

DEFINING CHARACTERISTICS

Major (Must Be Present)

Verbalization of nonacceptance of health status change or inability to be involved in problem solving or goal setting

Minor (May Be Present)

Lack of movement toward independence; extended period of shock, disbelief, or anger regarding health status change; lack of future-oriented thinking

ETIOLOGICAL, CONTRIBUTING, RISK FACTORS

Adjustment impairment can result from a variety of situations and health problems. Some common sources are listed below.

Pathophysiological

Spinal cord injury
Paralysis
Loss of limb
Cerebrovascular accident (CVA)
Myocardial infarction
Progressive neurological diseases
Cancer
Chronic obstructive pulmonary disease (COPD)

Treatment-related

Dialysis

Situational (Personal, Environmental)

Inadequate support systems
Unavailable support systems
Impaired cognition
Depression
Loss (object, person, job)
Divorce

Maturational

Child/adolescent
   Chronic disease
   Disability
Adult
   Loss of ability to practice vocation
   Role reversal
Elderly
   Normal physiological aging changes

Anxiety

DEFINITION

Anxiety: The state in which an individual/group experiences feelings of uneasiness (apprehension) and activation of the autonomic nervous system in response to a vague, nonspecific threat.

> **Author's Note:**
> Anxiety differs from fear in that the anxious person cannot identify the threat. With fear, the threat can be identified. Anxiety can be present without fear, but they usually coexist.

DEFINING CHARACTERISTICS

Major (Must Be Present)

Manifested by symptoms from three categories—physiological, emotional, and cognitive. Symptoms vary according to the level of anxiety.

Physiological

Increased heart rate   Voice tremors/pitch
Insomnia   changes

Elevated blood pressure
Fatigue and weakness
Increased respiratory rate
Flushing or pallor
Diaphoresis
Dry mouth
Dilated pupils
Body aches and pains (especially chest, back, neck)
Trembling
Restlessness
Palpitations
Faintness/dizziness
Nausea and/or vomiting
Paresthesias
Frequent urination
Hot and cold flashes
Diarrhea

Emotional

Person states that he has feelings of
Apprehension
Lack of self-confidence
Helplessness
Losing control
Nervousness
Tension, or being "keyed up"
Fear
Inability to relax
Unreality
Anticipation of misfortune
Person exhibits
Irritability/impatience
Criticism of self and others
Angry outbursts
Withdrawal
Crying
Lack of initiative
Tendency to blame others
Self-deprecation
Startle reaction

Cognitive

Inability to concentrate
Lack of awareness of surroundings
Forgetfulness
Rumination
Orientation to past rather than to present or future
Blocking of thoughts (inability to remember)
Hyperattentiveness

ETIOLOGICAL, CONTRIBUTING, RISK FACTORS

Pathophysiological

Any factor that interferes with the basic human needs for food, air, and comfort

Situational (Personal, Environmental)

Actual or perceived threat to self-concept
Change in status
and prestige
Failure (or success)
Lack of recognition
from others

Loss of valued
possessions
Ethical dilemmas

Actual or perceived loss of significant others
Death
Divorce
Cultural pressures

Moving
Temporary or
permanent
separation

Actual or perceived threat to biological integrity
Dying
Assault

Invasive procedures
Disease

Actual or perceived change in environment
Hospitalization
Moving
Retirement

Safety hazards
Environmental
pollutants

Actual or perceived change in socioeconomic
status
Unemployment
New job

Promotion

Transmission of another person's anxiety to the
individual

Maturational (Threat to Developmental Task)

Infant/child
Separation
Mutilation
Peer relationships
Achievement
Adolescent
Sexual development
Peer relationships
Independence

Adult
    Pregnancy
    Parenting
    Career development
    Effects of aging
Elderly
    Sensory losses
    Motor losses
    Financial problems
    Retirement

Body Temperature, Potential Altered

Hypothermia

Hyperthermia

Thermoregulation, Ineffective

Author's Note:

These diagnostic categories represent two different thermal problems. Potential Altered Body Temperature describes an individual at risk for an abnormal body temperature because of disease and treatments, *e.g.*, infection, surgery. The nursing interventions would focus on comfort measures and maintaining hydration. Hypothermia and Hyperthermia are abnormal temperature states that are treatable by nursing interventions by correcting the external causes, *e.g.*, inappropriate clothing, exposure to the elements (heat, cold), dehydration. The nursing focus for hypothermia and hyperthermia is prevention. I rec-
(Continued)

Author's Note (Continued)

ommend that these diagnoses be utilized as Potential Hyperthermia and Potential Hypothermia to more appropriately describe the nursing role. Severe hypothermia and hyperthermia are life-threatening situations and require medical and nursing interventions for treatment. Such situations are collaborative problems and should be labeled Potential Complication: Hypothermia or Hyperthermia.

DEFINITION

Potential Altered Body Temperature: The state in which an individual is at risk of failing to maintain body temperature within normal range because of internal factors.

DEFINING CHARACTERISTICS

Major (Must Be Present)

Presence of risk factors (see Etiological, Contributing, Risk Factors)

ETIOLOGICAL, CONTRIBUTING, RISK FACTORS

Pathophysiological

Illness or trauma affecting temperature regulation
Coma/increased intracranial pressure
Brain tumor/hypothalamic tumor/head trauma
Cerebrovascular accident (CVA)
Infection
Integument (skin) injury
Anemia
Neurovascular disease/peripheral vascular disease
Pheochromocytoma (tumor of the adrenal medulla)
Altered metabolic rate

Treatment-related

Medications (*e.g.*, vasodilators/vasoconstrictors)
Sedation
Parenteral fluid infusion/blood transfusion
Dialysis
Surgery

Maturational

Extremes of age (*e.g.*, newborn, elderly)

Hypothermia

DEFINITION

Hypothermia: The state in which an individual has or is at risk for a sustained reduction of body temperature of below 35°C (95°F) orally or 36°C (96°F) rectally.

DEFINING CHARACTERISTICS*

Major (80%–100%)

Reduction in body temperature below 35°C
    (95°F) orally or 36°C (96°F) rectally
Cool skin
Pallor (moderate)
Shivering (mild)

Minor (50%–79%)

Mental confusion/drowsiness/restlessness
Decreased pulse and respiration
Cachexia/malnutrition

ETIOLOGICAL, CONTRIBUTING, RISK FACTORS

Situational (Personal, Environmental)

Exposure to heat, cold, rain, snow, wind
Inappropriate clothing for climate

---

* Adapted from Carroll SM: Hypothermia: A Clinical Validation Study. (Unpublished, 1987)

Poverty (inability to pay for shelter or heat)
Extremes of weight
Consumption of alcohol
Dehydration
Inactivity

Maturational

Extremes of age (*e.g.,* newborn, elderly)

Hyperthermia

DEFINITION

Hyperthermia: The state in which an individual has or is at risk for a sustained elevation of body temperature of greater than 37.8°C (100°F) orally or 38.8°C (101°F) rectally due to external factors.

DEFINING CHARACTERISTICS

Major (Must Be Present)

Temperature greater than 37.8°C (100°F) orally or 38.8°C (101°F) rectally

Minor (May Be Present)

Flushed skin
Warm to touch
Increased respiratory rate
Tachycardia
Shivering/goose pimples
Dehydration
Specific or generalized aches and pains (*e.g.,* headache)
Malaise/fatigue/weakness
Loss of appetite

ETIOLOGICAL, CONTRIBUTING, RISK FACTORS

Situational (Personal, Environmental)

Exposure to heat, sun
Inappropriate clothing for climate
Poverty
Extremes of weight
Dehydration

Inactivity or vigorous activity
Lack of knowledge

Maturational

Extremes of age (*e.g.,* newborn, elderly)

Thermoregulation, Ineffective

DEFINITION

Ineffective Thermoregulation: The state in which an individual experiences or is at risk of experiencing an inability to effectively maintain normal body temperature in the presence of adverse or changing external factors.

> **Author's Note:**
> This diagnostic category is indicated when the nurse can maintain or assist an individual to maintain a body temperature within normal limits by manipulating external factors (*e.g.,* clothing) and environmental conditions. Individuals who are at high risk for this diagnosis are the elderly and neonates. For individuals with temperature fluctuations due to disease, infections, or trauma, see Potential Altered Body Temperature.

DEFINING CHARACTERISTICS

Major (Must Be Present)

Temperature fluctuations related to limited metabolic compensatory regulation in response to environmental factors

ETIOLOGICAL, CONTRIBUTING, RISK FACTORS

Situational (Personal, Environmental)

Fluctuating environmental temperatures
Cold or wet articles (clothes, cribs, equipment)

Inadequate heating system
Inadequate housing
Wet body surface
Inadequate clothing for weather (excessive,
    insufficient)

Maturational

Neonate
    Large surface area relative to body mass
    Limited ability to produce heat (metabolic)
    Limited shivering ability
    Increased basal metabolism
Premature (same as neonate but more severe)
Elderly
    Decreased basal metabolism
    Loss of adipose tissue (limbs)

Bowel Elimination, Altered*

Constipation

Colonic Constipation

Perceived Constipation

Diarrhea

Bowel Incontinence

Author's Note:
Altered Bowel Elimination represents a broad category that is probably too broad for clinical use. It is
    (Continued)

* This diagnostic category is not on the NANDA list but has been included for clarity or usefulness.

Author's Note (Continued)
recommended that more specific categories be used
when possible. The three diagnostic categories relating
to constipation represent one general constipation
category and two specific types. The treatment of
colonic constipation differs from the treatment of
perceived constipation. Refer to Carpenito LJ: Nursing Diagnosis: Application to Clinical Practice, 3rd
ed. Philadelphia, JB Lippincott, 1989 for nursing interventions for all three categories.

DEFINITION

Altered Bowel Elimination: The state in which an
individual experiences or is at high risk of experiencing bowel dysfunction resulting in diarrhea or
constipation.

DEFINING CHARACTERISTICS

Major (Must Be Present)

Reports or demonstrates one or more of the
    following:
    Hard, formed stool
    Painful defecation
    Habitual use of laxatives/enemas
    Bowel movements less than three times
        weekly
    Loose, liquid stools
    Increased frequency (more than three times a
        day)

Minor (May Be Present)

Painful defecation	Anorexia
Abdominal discomfort	Urgency
Rectal fullness	Abdominal cramping
Headache	Increased or decreased
	bowel sounds

ETIOLOGICAL, CONTRIBUTING, RISK FACTORS

See Etiological, Contributing, Risk Factors under
Constipation and Diarrhea.

Constipation

DEFINITION

Constipation: The state in which an individual experiences or is at high risk of experiencing stasis of the large intestine, resulting in infrequent elimination and hard, dry feces.

DEFINING CHARACTERISTICS

Major (Must Be Present)

Hard, formed stool
and/or
Defecation occurs fewer than three times a week

Minor (May Be Present)

Decreased bowel sounds
Reported feeling of rectal fullness
Reported feeling of pressure in rectum
Straining and pain on defecation
Palpable impaction

ETIOLOGICAL, CONTRIBUTING, RISK FACTORS

Pathophysiological

Malnutrition
Sensory-motor disorders
   Spinal cord lesions   Cerebrovascular
   Spinal cord injury   accident (CVA, stroke)
                          Neurological diseases
Metabolic and endocrine disorders
   Anorexia nervosa   Hypothyroidism
   Obesity   Hyperparathyroidism
Ileus
Pain (upon defecation)
   Hemorrhoids
   Back injury
Decreased peristalsis related to hypoxia (cardiac, pulmonary)
Megacolon

Treatment-related

Drug side-effects
  Antacids
  Iron
  Barium
  Aluminum
  Aspirin
  Phenothiazines
  Calcium
  Anticholinergics
  Anesthetics
  Narcotics (codeine, morphine)
  Diuretics
  Antiparkinsonian agents
Surgery
Habitual laxative use

Situational (Personal, Environmental)

Immobility
Pregnancy
Stress
Lack of exercise
Irregular evacuation patterns
Cultural/health beliefs
Lack of privacy
Inadequate diet (lack of roughage/thiamine)
Dehydration
Fear of rectal or cardiac pain
Faulty appraisal dementia

Maturational

Infant
  Formula
Child
  Toilet training (reluctance to interrupt play)
Elderly
  Decreased motility of gastrointestinal tract

Colonic Constipation

DEFINITION

Colonic Constipation: The state in which an individual experiences or is at risk of experiencing a delay in passage of food residue resulting in dry, hard stool.

DEFINING CHARACTERISTICS*

Major (80%–100%)

Decreased frequency   Painful defecation
Hard, dry stool   Abdominal distention
Straining at stool

Minor (50%–79%)

Rectal pressure
Headache, appetite impairment
Abdominal pain

ETIOLOGICAL, CONTRIBUTING, RISK FACTORS

Pathophysiological

Malnutrition
Sensory-motor disorders
  Spinal cord lesions   Neurological
  Spinal cord injury   diseases
  Cerebrovascular
    accident (CVA,
    stroke)
Metabolic and endocrine disorders
  Anorexia nervosa   Hypothyroidism
  Obesity   Hyperpara-
                               thyroidism

Ileus
Decreased peristalsis related to hypoxia (cardiac,
    pulmonary)
Megacolon

Treatment-related

Drug side-effects
  Antacids   Anticholinergics
  Iron   Anesthetics
  Barium   Narcotics (codeine,
  Aluminum   morphine)
  Aspirin   Diuretics
  Phenothiazines   Antiparkinsonian
  Calcium   agents

* Adapted from McLane AM, McShane RE: Empirical validation of defining characteristics of constipation: A study of bowel elimination practices of healthy adults. In Hurley ME (ed): Classification of Nursing Diagnoses: Proceedings of the Sixth Conference, pp 448–455. St Louis, CV Mosby, 1986

Surgery
Habitual laxative use

Situational (Personal, Environmental)

Immobility
Pregnancy
Stress
Lack of exercise
Irregular evacuation
    patterns

Lack of privacy
Inadequate diet (lack
    of roughage/
    thiamine)
Dehydration
Fear of rectal or
    cardiac pain

Maturational

Infant
    Formula
Child
    Toilet training (reluctance to interrupt play)
Elderly
    Decreased motility of gastrointestinal tract

Perceived Constipation Related to: (Specify)

DEFINITION

Perceived Constipation: The state in which an individual self-prescribes the daily use of laxatives, enemas, and/or suppositories to ensure a daily bowel movement.

DEFINING CHARACTERISTICS*

Major (80%–100%)

Expectation of a daily bowel movement with the resulting overuse of laxatives, enemas, and suppositories
Expected passage of stool at the same time every day

* McLane A, McShane R: Empirical validation of defining characteristics of constipation: A study of bowel elimination practices of healthy adults. In Hurley ME (ed): Classification of Nursing Diagnoses: Proceedings of the Sixth Conference, pp 448–455. St Louis, CV Mosby, 1986

ETIOLOGICAL, CONTRIBUTING, RISK FACTORS

Pathophysiological

Altered affect caused by change in
    Body chemistry
    Tumor
Obsessive-compulsive disorders
Central nervous system deterioration

Situational (Personal, Environmental)

Cultural/family health beliefs
Faulty appraisal

Diarrhea

DEFINITION

Diarrhea: The state in which an individual experiences or is at high risk of experiencing frequent passage of liquid stool or unformed stool.

DEFINING CHARACTERISTICS

Major (Must Be Present)

Loose, liquid stools
and/or
Increased frequency

Minor (May Be Present)

Urgency
Cramping/abdominal pain
Increased frequency of bowel sounds
Increase in fluidity or volume of stools

ETIOLOGICAL, CONTRIBUTING, RISK FACTORS

Pathophysiological

Nutritional disorders and malabsorptive
    syndromes

Kwashiorkor	Crohn's disease
Gastritis	Lactose intolerance
Peptic ulcer	Spastic colon
Diverticulitis	Celiac disease
Ulcerative colitis	(sprue)
	Irritable bowel

Metabolic and endocrine disorders
  Diabetes mellitus   Thyrotoxicosis
  Addison's disease
Dumping syndrome
Infectious process
  Trichinosis   Shigellosis
  Dysentery   Typhoid fever
  Cholera   Infectious hepatitis
  Malaria
Cancer
Uremia
Tuberculosis
Arsenic poisoning
Fecal impaction

Treatment-related

Surgical intervention of the bowel
  Loss of bowel   Ileal bypass
Drug side-effects
  Thyroid agents   Antibiotics
  Antacids   Cancer chemo-
  Laxatives   therapeutic
  Stool softeners   agents
Tube feedings

Bowel Incontinence

DEFINITION

Bowel Incontinence: The state in which an individual experiences a change in normal bowel habits characterized by involuntary passage of stool.

Author's Note:

This diagnostic category represents a situation in which nurses have multiple responsibilities. Individuals experiencing Bowel Incontinence have various responses that disrupt functioning, such as

Fear related to embarrassment over lack of control of bowels

Potential Impaired Skin Integrity related to irritative nature of feces on skin

I recommend that the nurse not use Bowel Incontinence but instead another diagnostic category that better describes the situation.

DEFINING CHARACTERISTICS

Major (Must Be Present)

Involuntary passage of stool

ETIOLOGICAL, CONTRIBUTING, RISK FACTORS

Pathophysiological

Loss of sphincter control
Progressive dementia
Progressive neuromuscular disorder, *e.g.,*
    multiple sclerosis
Inflammatory bowel disease

Situational

Depression
Cognitive impairment
Surgery
    Colostomy

Breastfeeding, Ineffective

DEFINITION

Ineffective Breastfeeding: The state in which a mother, infant, or child experiences or is at risk of experiencing dissatisfaction or difficulty with the breastfeeding process.

DEFINING CHARACTERISTICS

Major (Must Be Present)

Actual or perceived inadequate milk supply
Infant's inability to attach correctly onto
    maternal breast
No observable signs of oxytocin release

Observable signs of inadequate infant intake
Nonsustained suckling at the breast
Insufficient emptying of each breast at each
     feeding
Persistence of sore nipples beyond the first week
     of breastfeeding
Insufficient opportunity for suckling at the breast
Infant exhibiting fussiness and crying within the
     first hour after breastfeeding; unresponsive
     to other comfort measures
Infant arching and crying at the breast, resisting
     latching on

ETIOLOGICAL, CONTRIBUTING, RISK FACTORS

Pathophysiological

Mastitis
Breast anomaly
     inverted nipple(s)
Pain (breast, perineum, uterus)

Treatment-related

Previous breast surgery

Situational (Personal, Environmental)

History of breastfeeding difficulties/failure
Ambivalence (maternal, family)
Anxiety
Nonsupportive partner/family
Lack of knowledge
Interruption in breastfeeding
     Ill mother   Excess artificial
     Ill infant   nipple
     Work schedule   supplements

Maturational

Neonate/infant
     Prematurity
     Poor sucking reflex

Cardiac Output, Altered: Decreased: (Specify)

DEFINITION

Altered Cardiac Output: Decreased: The state in which an individual experiences a reduction in the amount of blood pumped by the heart, resulting in compromised cardiac function.

Author's Note:

This diagnostic category represents a situation in which nurses have multiple responsibilities. Individuals experiencing decreased cardiac output may present various responses that disrupt functioning, such as:

Activity Intolerance
Sleep Pattern Disturbance

Or they may be at risk for developing physiological complications, such as:

Dysrhythmias
Cardiogenic shock
Congestive heart failure

I recommend that the nurse not use Altered Cardiac Output: Decreased but instead select another diagnostic category that better describes the situation. (Refer to Activity Intolerance.)

It is also recommended that the physiological complications for which nurses monitor in individuals with decreased cardiac output, and for which they collaborate with medicine for treatment, be labeled collaborative problems, such as

Potential Complications:
Dysrhythmias
Cardiogenic shock
Hypoxia

(Continued)

DEFINING CHARACTERISTICS

Low blood pressure	Dysrhythmia
Rapid pulse	Oliguria
Restlessness	Fatigability
Cyanosis	Vertigo
Dyspnea	Edema (peripheral,
Angina	sacral)

Comfort, Altered*

Pain

Acute Pain*

Chronic Pain

Pruritus

Nausea/Vomiting

DEFINITION

Altered Comfort: The state in which an individual experiences an uncomfortable sensation in response to a noxious stimulus.

* This diagnostic category is not currently on the NANDA list but has been included for clarity and usefulness.

DEFINING CHARACTERISTICS

Major (Must Be Present)

The person reports or demonstrates a discomfort.

Minor (May Be Present)

> Autonomic response in acute pain
>> Blood pressure increased
>> Pulse increased
>> Respirations increased
>> Diaphoresis
>> Dilated pupils
> Guarded position
> Facial mask of pain
> Crying, moaning
> Abdominal heaviness
> Cutaneous irritation

ETIOLOGICAL, CONTRIBUTING, RISK FACTORS

Any factor can contribute to altered comfort. The
most common are listed below.

Pathophysiological

> Musculoskeletal disorders
>> Fractures   Arthritis

Contractures
Spasms
Visceral disorders
  Cardiac   Intestinal
  Renal   Pulmonary
  Hepatic
Cancer
Vascular disorders
  Vasospasm   Phlebitis
  Occlusion   Vasodilation
                  (headache)

Inflammation
  Nerve   Joint
  Tendon   Muscle
  Bursa
Contagious disease (rubella, chickenpox)

- Contractures
- Spasms
- Visceral disorders
  - Cardiac / Intestinal
  - Renal / Pulmonary
  - Hepatic
- Cancer
- Vascular disorders
  - Vasospasm / Phlebitis
  - Occlusion / Vasodilation (headache)
- Inflammation
  - Nerve / Joint
  - Tendon / Muscle
  - Bursa
- Contagious disease (rubella, chickenpox)

Treatment-related

Trauma (surgery, accidents)
  Diagnostic tests
    Venipuncture
    Invasive scanning (*e.g.,* intravenous
      pyelogram [IVP])
    Biopsy
  Medications

Situational (Personal, Environmental)

Immobility/improper positioning
Overactivity
Pressure points (tight cast, elastic bandage)
Pregnancy (prenatal, intrapartum, postpartum)
Allergic response
Chemical irritants
Stress

Pain

DEFINITION

Pain: The state in which an individual experiences and reports the presence of severe discomfort or an uncomfortable sensation.

Author's Note:
This diagnostic category represents an individual who is experiencing pain. Clinically, it is more useful to differentiate acute pain from chronic pain in order to prescribe nursing interventions. Refer to *Acute Pain* or *Chronic Pain* for specific nursing interventions.

DEFINING CHARACTERISTICS

Subjective
Communication (verbal or coded) of pain descriptors
Objective
Guarding behavior, protective
Self-focusing
Narrowed focus (altered time perception, withdrawal from social contact, impaired thought processes)
Distraction behavior (moaning, crying, pacing, seeking out other people and/or activities, restlessness)
Facial mask of pain (lackluster eyes, "beaten look," fixed or scattered movement, grimace)
Altered muscle tone (may span from listless to rigid)
Autonomic responses not seen in chronic stable pain (diaphoresis, blood pressure and pulse change, pupillary dilation, increased or decreased respiratory rate)

Acute Pain

DEFINITION

Acute Pain: The state in which an individual experiences pain that can last from one second to as long as six months. It subsides with healing or when the stimulus is removed.

DEFINING CHARACTERISTICS

Major (Must Be Present)

The person reports or exhibits pain (may be the only sign of pain).

Minor (May Be Present)

Fear of pain
Inability to concentrate
Guarded positioning
Muscle spasm
Increase in pulse, blood pressure, and respiration
Evidence of inflammation (redness, heat, swelling)
Rubbing or pulling of body part
Tense body posture

Chronic Pain

DEFINITION

Chronic Pain: The state in which an individual experiences pain that is persistent or intermittent and lasts for more than six months.

DEFINING CHARACTERISTICS

Major (Must Be Present)

The person reports that pain has existed for more than six months (may be the only assessment data present).

Minor (May Be Present)

Discomfort
Anger, frustration, depression because of situation
Facial mask of pain
Anorexia, weight loss
Insomnia
Guarded movement
Muscle spasms
Redness, swelling, heat

Color changes in affected area
Reflex abnormalities

Pruritus

DEFINITION

Pruritus: The state in which an individual experiences an unpleasant, irritating cutaneous sensation of itching/burning that causes a desire to scratch.

DEFINING CHARACTERISTICS

See Altered Comfort.

Nausea/Vomiting

DEFINITION

Nausea: The state in which an individual experiences a sensation of abdominal heaviness and uneasiness with an inclination to vomit.

Author's Note:

Acute nausea/vomiting is always a state of discomfort but not always a nutritional problem. When nausea/vomiting is persistent, the diagnostic category of Altered Nutrition: Less Than Body Requirements related to nausea/vomiting would be indicated.

DEFINING CHARACTERISTICS

Major (Must Be Present)

Complains of "sickness of the stomach" or "queasiness" and an inclination to vomit

Minor (May Be Present)

Anorexia
Flushed or chills

Diaphoresis
Pallor
Increased salivation

ETIOLOGICAL, CONTRIBUTING, RISK FACTORS
Pathophysiological

Fever
Infections (viral, bacterial, parasitic)
    Gastrointestinal   Influenza
    Renal
CNS disorders
    Meniere's disease   Labyrinthitis
Increased intracranial pressure
Cardiac disorders
    Acute myocardial infarction
Gastrointestinal/hepatic disorders
    Hiatal hernia   Pancreatitis
    Cholelithiasis   Hepatitis
    Gastritis
Endocrine disorders
    Diabetic acidosis   Adrenal
                          insufficiency
Anorexia nervosa, bulimia
Electrolyte imbalance
Cancer (biliary, hepatic, pancreatic)

Treatment-related

Side-effects of medications (*e.g.,* corticosteroids,
    cardiac glycosides, opiates, narcotics,
    chemotherapy)
Radiation
Alcohol
Anesthesia

Situational (Personal, Environmental)

Pain
Noxious stimuli
    Odors   Sounds
    Sights   Tastes
Motion (car, airplane, boat)
Contaminated foods

Maturational

Child
  Fever
Childhood diseases (*e.g.,* measles)
Adolescent/adult
  Pregnancy

Communication, Impaired*

Communication, Impaired Verbal

DEFINITION

Impaired Communication: The state in which an individual experiences, or could experience, a decreased ability to send or receive messages (*i.e.,* has difficulty exchanging thoughts, ideas, or desires).

Author's Note:

This diagnostic category represents communication problems that involve both sending and receiving messages (talking and listening).

DEFINING CHARACTERISTICS

Major (Must Be Present)

Inappropriate or absent speech or response

Minor (May Be Present)

Stuttering
Slurring

* This diagnostic category is not currently on the NANDA list but has been included for clarity and usefulness.

Communication, Impaired

Problem in finding the correct word when
    speaking
Weak or absent voice
Decreased auditory comprehension
Deafness or inattention to noises or voices
Confusion
Inability to speak the dominant language of the
    culture

ETIOLOGICAL, CONTRIBUTING, RISK FACTORS

Pathophysiological

Cerebral impairment
    Expressive or receptive aphasia
    Cerebrovascular accident (CVA)
    Brain damage (*e.g.,* birth/head trauma
    Central nervous system (CNS) depression/
        increased intracranial pressure
    Tumor (head, neck, or spinal cord)
    Mental retardation
    Chronic hypoxia/decreased cerebral blood
        flow
Neurologic impairment
    Quadriplegia
    Nervous system diseases (*e.g.,* myasthenia
        gravis, multiple sclerosis)
    Vocal cord paralysis
    Auditory nerve damage
Respiratory impairment (*e.g.,* shortness of
    breath)
Auditory impairment (decreased hearing)
Laryngeal edema/infection

Treatment-related

Surgery
    Endotracheal intubation
    Tracheostomy/tracheotomy/laryngectomy
    Surgery of the head, face, neck, or mouth
    Pain (especially of the mouth or throat)
    Drugs (*e.g.,* central nervous system [CNS]
        depressants, anesthesia)

Situational (Personal, Environmental)

Fatigue (affecting ability to listen)
No access to hearing aid/malfunction of hearing
     aid
Oral deformities
   Cleft lip or palate
   Malocclusion or fractured jaw
   Missing teeth
Speech pathology
   Stuttering
   Lisping
   Ankyloglossia ("tongue-tied")
   Voice problems
Language barrier (unfamiliar language or dialect)
Psychological barrier (*e.g.,* fear, shyness)
Lack of privacy
Lack of support system
Loss of recent memory recall

Maturational

Elderly (auditory losses)
Infant
Child

Communication, Impaired Verbal

DEFINITION

Impaired Verbal Communication: The state in which an individual experiences, or could experience, a decreased ability or inability to speak but can understand others.

DEFINING CHARACTERISTICS

Major (Must Be Present)

Inability to speak words but can understand
     others
or
Articulation or motor planning deficits

Minor (May Be Present)

Shortness of breath

ETIOLOGICAL, CONTRIBUTING, RISK FACTORS

See Impaired Communication.

Coping, Ineffective Individual

Defensive Coping

Ineffective Denial

DEFINITION

Ineffective Individual Coping: The state in which an individual experiences or is at risk of experiencing an inability to manage internal or environmental stressors adequately because of inadequate resources (physical, psychological, behavioral, and/or cognitive).

Author's Note:

This diagnostic category can be used to describe a variety of situations in which an individual does not adapt effectively to stressors. Examples can be isolating behaviors, aggression, and destructive behavior. If the response is inappropriate use of the defense mechanisms denial or defensiveness, the diagnosis Ineffective Denial or Defensive Coping can be used instead of Ineffective Individual Coping.

DEFINING CHARACTERISTICS*

Major (Must Be Present)

Change in usual communication patterns (if
    acute)
Verbalization of inability to cope
or
Inappropriate use of defense mechanisms
or
Inability to meet role expectations

Minor (May Be Present)

Anxiety
Reported life stress
Inability to problem-solve
Alteration in social participation
Destructive behavior toward self or others
High incidence of accidents
Frequent illnesses
Verbalization of inability to ask for help
Verbal manipulation
Inability to meet basic needs

ETIOLOGICAL, CONTRIBUTING, RISK FACTORS

Pathophysiological

Changes in body integrity
    Loss of body part
    Disfigurement secondary to trauma
Altered affect caused by changes in
    Body chemistry
    Tumor (brain)
    Intake of mood-altering substance
Physiological manifestations of persistent stress

Situational (Personal, Environmental)

Changes in physical environment
    War   Seasonal work
    Natural disaster   (migrant
    Relocation   worker)
                           Poverty

* Adapted from Vincent KG: The validation of a nursing
diagnosis. Nurs Clin North Am 20(4):631–639, 1985

Disruption of emotional bonds due to
- Death
- Separation or divorce
- Desertion
- Relocation
- Incarceration

Unsatisfactory support system

Institutionalization
- Jail
- Foster home
- Orphanage
- Educational institution
- Maintenance institution for the disabled

Sensory overload
- Factory environment
- Urbanization: crowding, noise pollution, excessive activity

Inadequate psychological resources
- Poor self-esteem
- Excessive negative beliefs about self
- Helplessness
- Lack of motivation to respond

Culturally related conflicts with life experiences
- Premarital sex
- Abortion

Maturational

Child
- Developmental tasks (independence vs. dependence)
- Entry into school
- Competition among peers
- Peer relationships

Adolescent
- Physical and emotional changes
- Independence from family
- Heterosexual relationships
- Sexual awareness
- Educational demands
- Career choices

Young adult
- Career choices
- Educational demands
- Leaving home
- Marriage
- Parenthood

Middle adult
- Physical signs of aging
- Problems with relatives

Career pressures
Child-rearing
problems
Elderly
Physical changes
Changes in financial
status
Changes in
residence

Social status needs
Aging parents

Retirement
Response of others
to older people

Treatment-related

Separation from family and home (*e.g.,*
hospitalization, confinement to a nursing
home)
Need for medical treatment conflicts with beliefs
Disfigurement due to surgery
Altered appearance due to drugs, radiation, or
other treatment
Altered affect due to hormonal therapy
Sensory overload due to medical technology
(*e.g.,* critical care units)

Defensive Coping

DEFINITION

Defensive Coping: The state in which an individual
repeatedly projects a falsely positive self-evaluation
as a defense against underlying perceived threats to
positive self-regard.

DEFINING CHARACTERISTICS*

Major (80%–100%)

Denial of obvious problems/weaknesses
Projection of blame/responsibility
Rationalizes failures

* Norris J, Kunes-Connell M: Self esteem disturbance: A
clinical validation study. In McLane A (ed): Classification
of Nursing Diagnoses: Proceedings of the Seventh Conference. St Louis, CV Mosby, 1987

Hypersensitive to slight criticism
Grandiosity

Minor (50%–79%)

Superior attitude toward others
Difficulty in establishing/maintaining
    relationships
Hostile laughter or ridicule of others
Difficulty in testing perceptions against reality
Lack of follow-through or participation in
    treatment or therapy

ETIOLOGICAL, CONTRIBUTING, RISK FACTORS

See Chronic Low Self-esteem.

Ineffective Denial

DEFINITION

Ineffective Denial: The state is which an individual minimizes or disavows symptoms or a situation to his/her detriment of health.

Author's Note:

This type of denial differs from the denial in response to a loss. The denial in response to an illness or loss is necessary to maintain psychological equilibrium and is beneficial. Ineffective Denial is not beneficial when the individual will not participate in regimens to improve health or the situation, *e.g.,* denial of substance abuse. If the cause of the ineffective denial is not known, Ineffective Denial related to unknown etiology can be used; for example, Ineffective Denial related to unknown etiology as manifested by repetitive refusal to admit that barbiturate use is a problem.

DEFINING CHARACTERISTICS*

Major (80%–100%)

Delays seeking or refuses health care attention to the detriment of health

Does not perceive personal relevance of symptoms or danger

Minor (50%–79%)

Uses home remedies (self-treatment) to relieve symptoms

Does not admit fear of death or invalidism

Minimizes symptoms

Displaces source of symptoms to other areas of the body

Unable to admit impact of disease on life pattern

Makes dismissive gestures or comments when speaking of distressing events

Displaces fear of impact of the condition

Displays inappropriate affect

ETIOLOGICAL, CONTRIBUTING, RISK FACTORS

Pathophysiological

Any chronic and/or terminal illness

Treatment-related

Prolonged treatment with no positive results

Situational/Psychological

Loss of job

Loss of spouse/significant other

Financial crisis

Feelings of negative self-concept, inadequacy, guilt, loneliness, despair, failure

Feelings of increased anxiety/stress, need to escape personal problems, anger, and frustration

* Norris J, Kunes-Connell M: Self esteem disturbance: A clinical validation study. In McLane A (ed): Classification of Nursing Diagnoses: Proceedings of the Seventh Conference. St Louis, CV Mosby, 1987

Feelings of omnipotence
Culturally permissive attitudes toward alcohol/
    drug use
Religious sanctions

Maturational

Adolescent
  Peer pressure
Adult
  Job stress
  Expectation of alcohol/drug use
  Losses (job, spouse, children)
Elderly
  Losses (spouse, function, financial)
  Retirement

Biological/Genetic

Family history of alcoholism

Coping: Potential for Growth, Family

DEFINITION

Family Coping: Potential for Growth. Effective management of adaptive tasks by a family member involved with the client's health challenge, who now is exhibiting the desire and readiness for enhanced health and growth in regard to self and in relation to the client.

Author's Note:

This diagnostic category describes components that are found in Altered Family Processes and Health-Seeking Behaviors. Until clinical research differentiates the category from the preceding ones, use Altered Family Processes or Health-Seeking Behaviors, depending on the data presented.

DEFINING CHARACTERISTICS

Family member attempts to describe the growth impact of a crisis on his or her own values, priorities, goals, or relationships

Family member moves in the direction of a health-promoting and enriching life-style that supports and monitors maturational processes, audits and negotiates treatment programs, and generally chooses experiences that optimize wellness

Individual expresses interest in making contact on a one-to-one basis or in a mutual-aid group with another person who has experienced a similar situation

ETIOLOGICAL, CONTRIBUTING, RISK FACTORS

See Health Seeking Behaviors and Altered Family Processes.

Coping: Compromised, Ineffective Family

DEFINITION

Ineffective Family Coping: Compromised: The state in which a usually supportive primary person (family member or close friend) is providing insufficient, ineffective, or compromised support, comfort, assistance, or encouragement that may be needed by the client to manage or master adaptive tasks related to his or her health challenge.

Author's Note:

This diagnostic category describes situations that are similar to the diagnostic categories Impaired Ad-
(*Continued*)

Author's Note (Continued)
justment and Altered Family Processes. Until clinical research differentiates this category from the preceding ones, use Impaired Adjustment and/or Altered Family Processes.

DEFINING CHARACTERISTICS

Subjective

Client expresses or confirms a concern or complaint about a significant other's response to his or her health problem

Significant person describes preoccupation with personal reactions, *e.g.,* fear, anticipatory grief, guilt, anxiety, to client's illness, disability, or other situational or developmental crises

Significant person describes or confirms an inadequate understanding or knowledge base that interferes with effective assistive or supportive behaviors

Objective

Significant person attempts assistive or supportive behaviors with less than satisfactory results

Significant person withdraws or enters into limited or temporary personal communication with the client at times of need

Significant person displays protective behavior disproportionate (too little or too much) to the client's abilities or need for autonomy

ETIOLOGICAL, CONTRIBUTING, RISK FACTORS

See Altered Family Processes.

Coping: Disabling, Ineffective Family

DEFINITION

Ineffective Family Coping: Disabling The state in which a family demonstrates destructive behavior in response to an inability to manage internal or external stressors due to inadequate resources (physical, psychological, cognitive, and/or behavioral).

Author's Note:

The diagnostic category Ineffective Family Coping: Disabling describes a family that has a history of demonstrating destructive overt or covert behavior or has adapted detrimentally to a stressor. This category differs from Altered Family Processes, which describes a family that usually functions constructively but is challenged by a stressor that has altered or may alter its functioning. Sustained Altered Family Processes may progress to Ineffective Family Coping.

DEFINING CHARACTERISTICS

Major (Must Be Present)

Neglectful care of the client
Decisions/actions that are detrimental to
    economic and/or social well-being
Neglectful relationships with other family
    members

Minor (May Be Present)

Distortion of reality regarding the client's health
problem
Intolerance
Rejection
Abandonment
Desertion
Psychosomaticism
Taking on illness signs of client
Agitation
Depression
Aggression
Hostility
Impaired restructuring of a meaningful life for
self
Prolonged overconcerns for client
Client's development of helpless inactive
dependence

ETIOLOGICAL, CONTRIBUTING, RISK FACTORS

The following describes those individuals or families
who are at high risk for contributing to a family's
destructive coping behavior.

Parent(s)
Single
Adolescent
Abusive
Emotionally
disturbed
Alcoholic

Drug addicted
Terminally ill
Acutely disabled/
accident victim
Elderly dependent

Child
Of unwanted
pregnancy
Of undesired gender
or of forced
intercourse
With undesired
characteristics

Physically
handicapped
Mentally
handicapped
Hyperactive
Terminally ill
Adolescent rebellion

Pathophysiological
Any condition that challenges one's ability for
self-care, for fulfilling role responsibilities,
and for financial independence can

contribute to Ineffective Family Coping.
See Altered Family Process for specific
situations.

Other

History of ineffective relationship with own
parents
History of abusive relationships with parents
Unrealistic expectations of child by parent
Unrealistic expectations of self by parent
Unrealistic expectations of parent by child
Unmet psychosocial needs of child by parent
Unmet psychosocial needs of parent by child

Decisional Conflict

DEFINITION

Decisional Conflict: The state in which an individual/
group experiences uncertainty about course of action
when the choice involves risk, loss, or challenge.

DEFINING CHARACTERISTICS*

Major (80%–100%)

Verbalized uncertainty about choices
Verbalization of undesired consequences of
alternative actions being considered
Vacillation between alternative choices
Delayed decision making

Minor (50%–79%)

Verbalized feeling of distress while attempting a
decision
Self-focusing
Physical signs of distress or tension (increased
heart rate, increased muscle tension,
restlessness, etc.) whenever the decision
comes within focus of attention

* Hiltunen E: Diagnostic content validity of the nursing
diagnosis: Decisional Conflict. Unpublished raw data, 1987

Questioning personal values and beliefs while attempting to make a decision

ETIOLOGICAL, CONTRIBUTING, RISK FACTORS

Many situations can contribute to decisional conflict, particularly those that involve complex medical interventions of great risk. Any decisional situation can precipitate conflict for an individual; thus, the examples listed below are not exhaustive but reflective of situations that may be problematic and possess factors that increase the difficulty.

Treatment-related

Surgery
   Tumor removal   Cosmetic
   Cataract   Joint replacement
   Laminectomy   Hysterectomy
   Orchiectomy   Transplant
Diagnostics
   Amniocentesis   X-rays
   Ultrasound
Chemotherapy
Radiation
Dialysis
Mechanical ventilation
Enteral feedings
Intravenous hydration

Situational

Personal
   Marriage   Institutionalization
   Separation   (child, parent)
   Divorce   Breast vs bottle
   Parenthood   feeding
   Birth control   Abortion
   Artificial   Sterilization
      insemination   Nursing home
   Adoption   placement
   Foster home
     placement

Work/Task
    Career change   Business
    Relocation   investments
                          Professional ethics
Lack of relevant information
Confusing information
Disagreement within support systems
Inexperience with decision making
Unclear personal values/beliefs
Conflict with personal values/beliefs
Resignation
Family history of poor prognosis
Hospital environment—loss of control
Ethical dilemmas
    Quality of life
    Cessation of life-support systems
    "Do not resuscitate" orders

Maturational

Adolescent
    Peer pressure   Whether to
    Sexual activity   continue a
    Alcohol/drug use   relationship
    Illegal/dangerous   College
        situations   Career choice
    Use of birth control
Adult
    Career change   Parenthood
    Marriage
Older adult
    Retirement   Nursing home
                    placement

Disuse Syndrome: Potential for

DEFINITION

Potential for Disuse Syndrome: The state in which an individual is at risk for deterioration of body systems as a result of musculoskeletal inactivity.

DEFINING CHARACTERISTICS

Presence of risk factors (see Etiological, Contributing, Risk Factors)

ETIOLOGICAL, CONTRIBUTING, RISK FACTORS

Pathophysiological

Decreased sensorium
Unconsciousness
Neuromuscular impairment
  Multiple sclerosis   Muscular dystrophy
  Parkinsonism   Partial or total
  Gullain-Barré   paralysis
    syndrome   Spinal cord injury
Musculoskeletal conditions
  Fractures   Rheumatic diseases
End-stage disease
  Acquired immuno-   Renal disease
    deficiency   Cardiac disease
    syndrome   Cancer
    (AIDS)
Psychiatric/mental health disorders
  Major depression   Severe phobias
  Catatonic state

Treatment-related

Surgery (amputation, skeletal)
Traction/casts/splints
Prescribed immobility
Mechanical ventilation
Invasive vascular lines

Situational

Depression   Debilitated state
Fatigue   Pain

Maturational

Newborn/infant/child/adolescent
  Down Syndrome
  Legg-Calvé-Perthes   Osteogenesis
    Disease   imperfecta
  Cerebral palsy

Spina bifida	Autism
Risser turnbuckle jacket	Mental/physical disability
Juvenile arthritis	
Elderly	
Decreased motor agility	Muscle weakness
	Presenile dementia

Diversional Activity Deficit

DEFINITION

Diversional Activity Deficit: The state in which an individual or group experiences or is at risk of experiencing decreased stimulation from or interest in leisure activities.

DEFINING CHARACTERISTICS

Major (Must Be Present)

Observed on statements of boredom/depression from inactivity

Minor (May Be Present)

Constant expression of unpleasant thoughts or feelings
Yawning or inattentiveness
Flat facial expression
Body language (shifting of body away from speaker)
Restlessness/fidgeting
Immobile (on bed rest or confined)
Weight loss or gain
Hostility

ETIOLOGICAL, CONTRIBUTING, RISK FACTORS

Pathophysiological

Communicable disease
Pain

Treatment-related

Long or frequent treatments

Situational (Personal, Environmental)

No peers or friends
Monotonous environment
Long-term hospitalization or confinement
Lack of motivation
Loss of ability to perform usual or favorite
   activities
Excessive long hours of stressful work
No time for leisure activities
Career changes (*e.g.,* teacher to homemaker,
   retirement)
Children leaving home ("empty nest")
Immobility
Decreased sensory perception (*e.g.,* blindness,
   hearing loss)

Maturational

Infant/child
   Lack of appropriate toys/peers
Elderly
   Sensory-motor deficits

Dysreflexia

DEFINITION

Dysreflexia: The state in which an individual with a spinal cord injury at T7 or above experiences or is at risk for experiencing uninhibited sympathetic response of the nervous system to a noxious stimulus.

> **Author's Note:**
> This is a situation that the nurse and/or client can prevent or treat. If the nurse's initial treatment does
> *(Continued)*

DEFINING CHARACTERISTICS

Major (Must Be Present)

Individual with spinal cord injury T7 or above with

Paroxysmal hypertension (sudden periodic elevated blood pressure in which systolic pressure is over 140 mm Hg and diastolic is above 90 mm Hg)

Bradycardia or tachycardia (pulse rate of less than 60 or more than 100 beats per minute)

Diaphoresis (above the injury)

Red splotches on the skin (above the injury)

Pallor (below the injury)

Headache (a diffuse pain in different portions of the head and not confined to any nerve distribution area)

Minor (May Be Present)

Chilling

Conjunctival congestion

Horner's syndrome (contraction of the pupil, partial ptosis of the eyelid, enophthalmos and sometimes loss of sweating over the affected side of the face

Paresthesia

Pilomotor reflex

Blurred vision

Chest pain

Metallic taste in the mouth

Nasal congestion

ETIOLOGICAL, CONTRIBUTING, RISK FACTORS

Pathophysiological

Visceral stretching and irritation
    Bowel
        Constipation   Fecal impaction
    Bladder
        Distended bladder   Infection
        Urinary calculi
Stimulation of skin (abdominal, thigh)
Acute abdominal condition
Spastic sphincter

Treatment-related

Removal of fecal impaction
Clogged or nonpatent catheter
Surgical incision

Situational (Personal, Environmental)

Lack of knowledge

Family Processes, Altered

DEFINITION

Altered Family Processes: The state in which a normally supportive family experiences a stressor that challenges its previously effective functioning ability.

Author's Note:

The nursing diagnosis Altered Family Processes describes a family that usually functions optimally but is challenged by a stressor that has altered or may *(Continued)*

DEFINING CHARACTERISTICS

Major (Must Be Present)

Family system cannot or does not
  Adapt constructively to crisis
  Communicate openly and effectively between
    family members

Minor (May Be Present)

Family system cannot or does not
  Meet physical needs of all its members
  Meet emotional needs of all its members
  Meet spiritual needs of all its members
  Express or accept a wide range of feelings
  Seek or accept help appropriately

ETIOLOGICAL, CONTRIBUTING, RISK FACTORS

Any factor can contribute to Altered Family Processes. Some common factors are listed below.

Pathophysiological

Illness of family member
  Discomforts related   Disabling
    to the   treatments
    symptoms of   Expensive
    the illness   treatments
  Change in the
    family
    member's
    ability to
    function

Time-consuming
      treatments
Trauma
   Surgery   Loss of body part or
                                     function

Treatment-related

Disruption of family routines due to time-
      consuming treatments (*e.g.,* home dialysis)
Physical changes due to treatments of ill family
      member
Emotional changes in all family members due to
      treatments of ill family member
Financial burden of treatments for ill family
      member
Hospitalization of ill family member

Situational (Personal, Environmental)

Loss of family member
   Death   Incarceration
   Going away to   Desertion
      school   Hospitalization
   Separation
   Divorce
Gain of family member
   Birth   Marriage
   Adoption   Elderly relative
Poverty
Disaster
Relocation
Economic crisis
   Unemployment   Financial loss
Change in family roles
   Working mother   Retirement
Birth of child with defect
Conflict
   Goal conflicts   Cultural conflict
   Moral conflict with   with reality
      reality   Personality conflict
                                     in family
Breach of trust between members
   Dishonesty
   Adultery
History of psychiatric illness in family

Social deviance by family member (including crime)

Fatigue

DEFINITION

Fatigue: The self-recognized state in which an individual experiences an overwhelming sustained sense of exhaustion and decreased capacity for physical and mental work that is not relieved by rest.

> **Author's Note:**
> Fatigue is different from tiredness. Tiredness is a transient, temporary state from lack of sleep, improper nutrition, sedentary life-style, or a temporary increase in work or social responsibilities. Fatigue is a pervasive, subjective, drained feeling that cannot be eliminated but that one can adapt to with assistance. Activity Intolerance is different from Fatigue in that the person with activity intolerance will be assisted to increase endurance to progress and increase his activity. The person with chronic fatigue will not return to the previous level of functioning.

DEFINING CHARACTERISTICS*

Major (80%–100%)

Verbalization of an unremitting and overwhelming lack of energy
Inability to maintain usual routines

* Voith AM, Frank AM, Pigg JS: Validations of fatigue as a nursing diagnosis. In McLane A (ed): Classification of Nursing Diagnoses: Proceedings of the Seventh National Conference, p 280. St Louis, CV Mosby, 1987

Minor (50%–79%)

Perceived need for additional energy to
accomplish routine tasks
Increase in physical complaints
Emotionally labile or irritable
Impaired ability to concentrate
Decreased performance
Lethargic or listless
Lack of interest in surroundings/introspection
Decreased libido
Accident prone

ETIOLOGICAL, CONTRIBUTING, RISK FACTORS

Many factors can cause fatigue, some common factors
are the following:

Pathophysiological

Acute infections
  Mononucleosis   Viruses
  Hepatitis
Fever
Chronic infection
  Hepatitis   Endocarditis
Impaired oxygen transport system
  Congestive heart   Anemia
    failure   Peripheral vascular
  Chronic obstructive   disease
    lung disease
Endocrine/metabolic disorders
  Diabetus Mellitus   Pituitary disorders
  Hypothyroidism   Addison's disease
Chronic diseases (*e.g.,* renal failure, cirrhosis)
Neuromuscular disorders
  Parkinson's disease   Myasthenia gravis
  Arthritis   Multiple sclerosis
Obesity
Electrolyte imbalances
Cancer
Nutritional disorders

Gait disorders
Acquired immunodeficiency syndrome (AIDS)

Treatment-related

Chemotherapy
Radiation therapy
Antidepressants
Drug withdrawal

Situational

Depression
Extreme stress
Crisis (personal, developmental, career, family,
    financial)
Sensory overload (noise, illumination, etc.)
Extreme temperatures
Prolonged excessive role demands

Maturational

Adult
    Pregnancy (first trimester)
    Caregiver (ill child, aging parent)

Fear

DEFINITION

Fear: The state in which an individual or group experiences a feeling of physiological or emotional disruption related to an identifiable source that is perceived as dangerous.

DEFINING CHARACTERISTICS

Major (Must Be Present)

Feelings of: dread, fright, apprehension
and/or
Behaviors of: avoidance, narrowing of focus on danger, and deficits in attention, performance, and control

Minor (May Be Present)

Verbal reports of: panic, obsessions
Behavioral acts of
   Aggression
   Escape
   Hypervigilance
   Dysfunctional immobility
   Compulsive mannerisms
   Increased questioning/verbalization
Visceral–somatic activity
   Musculoskeletal
      Muscle tightness
      Fatigue
   Cardiovascular
      Palpitations
      Rapid pulse
      Increased blood pressure
   Respiratory
      Shortness of breath
      Increased rate
   Gastrointestinal
      Anorexia
      Nausea/vomiting
      Diarrhea

Genitourinary
   Urinary frequency
Skin
   Flush/pallor
   Sweating
   Paresthesia
Central nervous system (CNS)/perceptual
   Syncope
   Insomnia
   Lack of concentration
   Irritability
   Absentmindedness
   Nightmares
   Dilated pupils

ETIOLOGICAL, CONTRIBUTING, RISK FACTORS

Fear can occur as a response to a variety of health problems, situations, or conflicts. Some common sources are indicated below.

Pathophysiological

Loss of body part
Loss of body function
Disabling illness
Long-term disability
Terminal disease

Treatment-related

Hospitalization
Surgery and its outcome
Anesthesia
Invasive procedures
Radiation

Situational (Personal, Environmental)

Influences of others
Pain
New environment
New people
Lack of knowledge
Change or loss of significant other
Divorce
Success
Failure

Maturational

Child
   Age-related fears (dark, strangers)
   Influence of others

Adolescent
   School adjustments
   Social and intellectual competitiveness
   Independence
   Authorities
Adult
   Marriage
   Pregnancy
   Parenthood
Elderly
   Retirement
   Relinquishing roles
   Functional losses

Fluid Volume Deficit

DEFINITION

Fluid Volume Deficit: The state in which an individual who is not NPO experiences or is at risk of experiencing vascular, interstitial, or intracellular dehydration.

Author's Note:
This diagnostic category represents situations in which nurses can prescribe definitive treatment to prevent fluid depletion or to reduce or eliminate contributing factors such as insufficient oral intake. Situations that represent hypovolemia caused by hemorrhage or NPO states should be considered collaborative problems, not nursing diagnoses. Nursing monitors to detect these situations and collaborates with medicine for treatment. These situations can be labeled Potential Complication: Hemorrhage, or Potential Complication: Hypovolemia.

DEFINING CHARACTERISTICS

Major (Must Be Present)

Output greater than intake
Dry skin/mucous membranes

Minor (May Be Present)

Increased serum sodium
Increased pulse rate (from baseline)
Decreased urine output or excessive urine output
Concentrated urine or urinary frequency
Decreased fluid intake
Decreased skin turgor
Thirst/nausea/anorexia

ETIOLOGICAL, CONTRIBUTING, RISK FACTORS

Pathophysiological

Excessive urinary output
   Uncontrolled diabetes
   Diabetes insipidus (inappropriate antidiuretic
      hormone)
Burns (post-acute)
Fever or increased metabolic rate
Infection
Abnormal drainage
   Wound
   Excessive menses
   Other
Peritonitis
Diarrhea

Situational (Personal, Environmental)

Vomiting/nausea
Decreased motivation to drink liquids
   Depression
   Fatigue
Dietary problems
   Fad diets/fasting
   Anorexia
   High-solute tube feedings

Difficulty swallowing or feeding self
  Oral pain
  Fatigue
Climate exposure
  Extreme heat/sun
  Extreme dryness
Hyperpnea
Extreme exercise effort/diaphoresis
Excessive use of
  Laxatives or enemas
  Diuretics or alcohol

Maturational

Infant/child
  Decreased fluid reserve
  Decreased ability to concentrate urine
Elderly
  Decreased fluid reserve
  Decreased sensation of thirst

Fluid Volume Excess

DEFINITION

Fluid Volume Excess: The state in which an individual experiences or is at risk of experiencing intracellular or interstitial fluid overload.

Author's Note:

This diagnostic category represents situations in which nursing can prescribe definitive treatment to reduce or eliminate factors that contribute to edema or can teach preventive actions. Situations that represent vascular fluid overload should be considered collaborative problems, not nursing diagnoses. They can be labeled Potential Complication: Congestive heart failure, or Potential Complication: Hypervolemia.

DEFINING CHARACTERISTICS

Major (Must Be Present)

Edema
Taut, shiny skin

ETIOLOGICAL, CONTRIBUTING, RISK FACTORS

Pathophysiological

Renal failure, acute or chronic
Decreased cardiac output
  Myocardial   Valvular disease
    infarction   Tachycardia/
  Congestive heart   arrhythmias
    failure
  Left ventricular
    failure
Varicosities of the legs
Liver disease
  Cirrhosis   Cancer
  Ascites
Tissue insult
  Injury to the cell   Hypoxia of the cell
    wall
Inflammatory process
Hormonal disturbances
  Pituitary   Estrogen
  Adrenal

Treatment-related

Corticosteroid therapy

Situational (Personal, Environmental)

Excessive sodium intake/fluid intake
Low protein intake
  Fad diets   Malnutrition
Dependent venous pooling/venostasis
  Immobility   Standing or sitting
                 for long periods
Venous pressure point
  Tight cast or bandage
Pregnancy
Inadequate lymphatic drainage

Maturational

Elderly (decreased cardiac output)

Grieving*

Grieving, Anticipatory

Grieving, Dysfunctional

DEFINITION

Grieving: The state in which an individual or group experiences an actual or perceived loss (person, object, function, status, relationship) or the state in which an individual or group responds to the realization of a future loss (anticipatory grieving).

> **Author's Note:**
> This diagnostic category represents individuals or groups that have sustained a loss. Since it may be problematic and hazardous to have to label Grieving as either anticipatory or dysfunctional, the Grieving category provides a useful alternative to describe individuals experiencing the normal process of grieving.

DEFINING CHARACTERISTICS

Major (Must Be Present)

The person
Reports an actual or perceived loss (person, object, function, status relationship)
or
Anticipates a loss

* This diagnostic category is not currently on the NANDA list but has been included for clarity or usefulness.

Minor (May Be Present)

Denial
Guilt
Anger
Despair
Feelings of
worthlessness
Suicidal thoughts
Crying
Sorrow
Hallucinations

Delusions
Phobias
Anergia
Inability to
concentrate
Visual, auditory, and
tactile
hallucinations
about the object
or person

ETIOLOGICAL, CONTRIBUTING, RISK FACTORS

Many situations can contribute to feelings of loss. Some common situations are listed below.

Pathophysiological

Loss of function (actual or potential) related to a
disorder
Neurological
Cardiovascular
Sensory
Musculoskeletal

Digestive
Respiratory
Renal

Loss of function or body part related to
Trauma

Treatment-related

Dialysis
Surgery (mastectomy, colostomy, hysterectomy)

Situational (Personal, Environmental)

Chronic pain
Terminal illness
Death
Changes in life-style
Childbirth
Marriage
Separation
Divorce

Child leaving home
(*e.g.,* college or
marriage)
Loss of career

Type of relationship (with the person who is
leaving or is gone)

Multiple losses or crises
Lack of social support system

Maturational

Loss associated with aging
Friends   Function
Occupation   Home

Grieving, Anticipatory

DEFINITION

Anticipatory Grieving: The state in which an individual/group experiences feelings in response to an expected significant loss.

DEFINING CHARACTERISTICS

Major (Must Be Present)

Expressed distress at potential loss

Minor (May Be Present)

Denial
Guilt
Anger
Sorrow
Change in eating habits
Change in sleep patterns
Change in social patterns
Change in communication patterns
Decreased libido

ETIOLOGICAL, CONTRIBUTING, RISK FACTORS

See Grieving.

Grieving, Dysfunctional

DEFINITION

Dysfunctional Grieving: The state in which an individual or group experiences prolonged unresolved grief and engages in detrimental activities.

DEFINING CHARACTERISTICS

Major (Must Be Present)

Unsuccessful adaptation to loss
Prolonged denial, depression
Delayed emotional reaction

Minor (May Be Present)

Social isolation or withdrawal
Failure to develop new relationships/interests
Failure to restructure life after loss

ETIOLOGICAL, CONTRIBUTING, RISK FACTORS

See Grieving.

Growth and Development, Altered

DEFINITION

Altered Growth and Development: The state in which an individual has or is at risk for an impaired ability to perform tasks of his/her age group or impaired growth.

Author's Note:

The focus of this category will be children and adolescents. When an adult has not accomplished a developmental task, the nurse should assess for the altered functioning that has resulted from the failure to meet a developmental task; for example, Impaired Social Interactions or Ineffective Individual Coping.

DEFINING CHARACTERISTICS

Major (Must Be Present)

Inability to perform or difficulty performing skills or behaviors typical of his/her age group; for example, motor, personal/social, language/cognition

and/or

Altered physical growth: Weight lagging behind height by two standard deviations; pattern of height and weight percentiles indicating a drop in pattern

Minor (May Be Present)

Inability to perform self-care or self-control activities appropriate for age

Flat affect, listlessness, decreased responses, slow in social responses, shows limited signs of satisfaction to caregiver, shows limited eye contact, difficulty feeding, decreased appetite, lethargic, irritable, negative mood, regression in self-toileting, regression in self-feeding

Infants: watchfulness, interrupted sleep pattern

ETIOLOGICAL, CONTRIBUTING, RISK FACTORS

Pathophysiological

Circulatory impairment
  Congenital heart defects
  Congestive heart failure

Neurological impairment
   Cerebral damage
   Congenital defects
   Cerebral palsy
   Microcephaly
Gastrointestinal impairment
   Malabsorption syndrome
   Gastroesophageal reflux
   Cystic fibrosis
Endocrine or renal impairment
   Hormonal disturbance
Musculoskeletal impairments
   Congenital anomalies of extremities
   Muscular dystrophy
Acute illness
Prolonged pain
Repeated acute illness, chronic illness
Inadequate caloric, nutritional intake

Treatment-related

Prolonged, painful treatments
Repeated or prolonged hospitalization
Traction or casts that alter locomotion
Prolonged bed rest
Isolation due to disease processes
Confinement for ongoing treatment

Situational (Personal, Environmental)

Parental lack of knowledge
Stress (acute, transient, or chronic)
Hospitalization or change in usual environment
Separation from significant others (parents,
     primary caregiver)
Inadequate, inappropriate parental support
     (neglect, abuse)
Inadequate sensory stimulation (neglect,
     isolation)
Parent–child conflict
School-related stressors
Maternal or parental anxiety
Loss of significant other
Loss of control over environment (established
     rituals, activities, established hours of
     contact with family)
Multiple caregivers

Maturational

Infant–toddler (birth to three years)
    Lack of stimulation
    Separation from parents/significant others
    Change in environment
    Restriction of activity
    Inadequate parental support
    Inability to trust significant other
    Inability to communicate (deafness)
Pre–school age (four to six years)
    Restriction of activity
    Loss of ability to communicate
    Lack of stimulation
    Lack of significant other
    Loss of significant other (death, divorce)
    Loss of peer group
    Loss of independence
    Fear of mutilation/pain/abandonment
    Removal from home environment
School age (six to eleven years)
    Loss of individual control
    Loss of significant other
    Loss of peer group
    Fear of immobility, mutilation, death
    Fear of intrusive procedures
    Strange environment
Adolescent (twelve to eighteen years)
    Loss of independence and autonomy
    Disruption of peer relationships
    Disruption in body image
    Interruption of intellectual achievement
    Loss of significant other

Health Maintenance, Altered

DEFINITION

Altered Health Maintenance: The state in which an individual or group experiences or is at risk of experiencing a disruption in health because of an un-

healthy life-style or lack of knowledge to manage a
condition.

> **Author's Note:**
> Altered Health Maintenance is a diagnostic category
> that can be used to describe a person or persons who
> desire to change an unhealthy life-style (obesity, to-
> bacco use) or who need teaching for self-management
> of a disease or condition.

DEFINING CHARACTERISTICS (in the Absence of Disease)

Major (Must Be Present)

Reports or demonstrates an unhealthy practice
or life-style
Reckless driving of vehicle
Substance abuse
Participation in high-risk activities (*e.g.,*
recreational: skydiving/scuba diving, hang
gliding; occupational: police, firefighting,
mining, etc.)
Presence of obvious behavior disorders
(compulsiveness, belligerence)
Overeating
Reports or demonstrates
Skin and nails
Malodorous
Unclean
Skin lesions
(pustules,
rashes, dry or
scaly skin)
Respiratory system
Frequent
infections
Chronic cough
Oral cavity
Frequent sores
(on tongue,

buccal
mucosa)
Loss of teeth at
early age
Sunburn
Unusual color,
pallor
Unexplained scars

Dyspnea with
exertion

Lesions associated
with lack of
oral care or
substance

abuse
(leukoplakia,
fistulas)

Gastrointestinal system and nutrition

Obesity

Anorexia

Cachexia

Chronic anemia

Chronic bowel
irregularity

Chronic dyspepsia

Musculoskeletal system

Frequent muscle strain, backaches, neck
pain

Diminished flexibility and muscle strength

Genitourinary system

Frequent venereal lesions and infections

Frequent use of potentially unhealthful
over-the-counter products (chemical
douches, perfumed vaginal products,
nasal sprays, etc.)

Constitutional

Chronic fatigue, malaise, apathy

Neurosensory

Presence of facial tics (nonconvulsant)

Headaches

Psychoemotional

Emotional fragility

Behavior disorders (compulsiveness,
belligerence)

Frequent feelings of being overwhelmed

ETIOLOGICAL, CONTRIBUTING, RISK FACTORS

A variety of factors can produce altered health maintenance. Some common causes are listed below.

Pathophysiological

Any new medical condition, regardless of the
severity of illness

Treatment-related

Lack of previous exposure
New or complex treatment

Situational (Personal, Environmental)

Lack of exposure to the experience
Language differences
Information misinterpretation
Personal characteristics

Lack of motivation	Ineffective coping patterns (*e.g.,* anxiety, depression, nonproductive denial of situation, avoidance coping)
Lack of education or readiness	

Changes in finances
Lack of access to adequate health care services
Inadequate health practice
External locus of control
Religious beliefs
Cultural beliefs

Maturational

Lack of education of age-related factors.
Examples include

Child

Sexuality and sexual development	Substance abuse
	Nutrition
Safety hazards	

Adolescent

Same as child	Substance abuse (alcohol, other drugs, tobacco)
Automobile safety practices	
	Health maintenance practices

Adult

Parenthood	Safety practices
Sexual function	Health maintenance practices

Elderly

Effects of aging	Sensory deficits

See table for age-related conditions.

Health Seeking Behaviors: (Specify)

DEFINITION

Health Seeking Behaviors: The state in which an individual in stable health actively seeks ways to alter personal health habits and/or the environment to move toward a higher level of wellness.*

Author's Note:

This diagnostic category can be used to describe the individual/family that desires health teaching related to the promotion and maintenance of health (preventive behavior, age-related screening, optimal nutrition, etc.). This diagnostic category should be used to describe an asymptomatic person. However, it can be used for a person with a chronic disease to help that person attain a higher level of wellness. For example, a woman with lupus erythematosus can have the diagnosis Health-seeking Behaviors: regular exercise program.

DEFINING CHARACTERISTICS

Major (Must Be Present)

Expressed or observed desire to seek information
    for health promotion

Minor (May Be Present)

Expressed or observed desire for increased
    control of health practice
Expression of concern about current
    environmental conditions on health status

* Stable health status is defined as follows: age-appropriate illness prevention measures are achieved; client reports good or excellent health; signs and symptoms of disease, if present, are controlled.

Stated or observed unfamiliarity with
community wellness resources
Demonstrated or observed lack of knowledge in
health promotion behaviors

Health Seeking Behaviors: (Specify)

ETIOLOGICAL, CONTRIBUTING, RISK FACTORS

Situational (Personal, Environmental)

Role changes
Marriage
Parenthood
"Empty-nest syndrome"
Retirement
Lack of knowledge of need for
Preventive behavior (disease)
Screening practices for age and risk
Optimal nutrition and weight control
Regular exercise program
Constructive stress management
Supportive social networks
Responsible role participation

Maturational

See table (Primary and Secondary Prevention for
Age-related Situations) on pages 77 through
83.

(Text continues on p 84.)

Primary and Secondary Prevention for Age-related Conditions

Developmental Level	Primary Prevention	Secondary Prevention

Infancy (0–1 year)	Parent education
	Infant safety
	Nutrition
	Breastfeeding
	Sensory stimulation
	Infant massage and touch
	Visual stimulation
	  Activity
	  Colors
	Auditory stimulation
	  Verbal
	  Music
	Immunizations
	DPT
	TOPV } at 2, 4, and 6 months
	Oral hygiene
	Teething biscuits
		Complete physical examination every 2–3 months
		Screening at birth
		  Congenital hip
		  Phenylketonuria (PKU)
		  Sickle cell disease
		  Cystic fibrosis
		  Vision (startle reflex)
		  Hearing (response to and localization of sounds)
		Tuberculin test at 12 months
		Developmental assessments
		Screen and intervene for high risk
		  Low birth weight
		  Maternal substance abuse during pregnancy
		  Alcohol: fetal alcohol syndrome
		  Cigarettes: sudden infant death syndrome (SIDS)
		  Drugs: addicted neonate
		  Maternal infections during pregnancy

(Continued)

77

Primary and Secondary Prevention for Age-related Conditions (Continued)

Developmental Level	Primary Prevention	Secondary Prevention
Preschool (1–5 years)	Fluoride Avoid sugared food and drink Parent education Teething Discipline Nutrition Accident prevention Normal growth and development Child education Dental self-care Dressing Bathing with assistance Feeding self-care Immunizations DPT } at 18 months TOPV } MMR at 15 months Dental/oral hygiene Fluoride treatments	Complete physical examination between 2 and 3 years and preschool (urinalysis, CBC) Tuberculin test at 3 years Developmental assessments (annual) Speech development Hearing Vision Screen and intervene Plumbism Developmental lag Neglect or abuse Strabismus Hearing deficit Vision deficit

Fluoridated water
Dietary counsel

School age
(6–11 years)

Health education of child
  "Basic 4" nutrition
  Accident prevention
  Outdoor safety
  Substance abuse counsel
  Anticipatory guidance for physical
    changes at puberty

Immunizations
  Tetanus, at 10 years
  DPT } Boosters between
  TOPV } 4 and 6 years

Professional dental hygiene every 6–12
  months
  Continue fluoridation
  Complete physical examination

Complete physical examination
Tuberculin test every 3 years (at ages 6 and 9)
Developmental measurements
  Language
  Vision: Snellen charts at school
    6–8 years, use "E" chart
    Over 8 years, use alphabet chart
  Hearing: audiogram

Adolescence
(12–19 years)

Health education
  Proper nutrition and healthful diets
  Sex education with family planning,
    male/female
  Safe driving skills

Complete physical examination (prepuberty or age 13)
Blood pressure
Cholesterol
Tuberculin test at 12 years
VDRL, CBC, urinalysis

(Continued)

79

Primary and Secondary Prevention for Age-related Conditions *(Continued)*

Developmental Level	Primary Prevention	Secondary Prevention
	Adult challenges	Female: breast self-examination
	Seeking employment and career choices	Male: testicular self-examination
	Dating and marriage	Female, if sexually active: Papanicolaou test and pelvic examination twice, one year apart (cervical examination), then gonorrhea culture with pelvic examination), then every 3 years if both are negative
	Confrontation with substance abuse	
	Safety in athletics	Screening and interventions if high risk
	Skin care	Depression
	Professional dental hygiene every 6–12 months	Suicide
		Substance abuse
	Immunization	Pregnancy
	Tetanus without trauma	Family history of alcoholism or domestic violence
	TOPV booster at 12–14 years	
Young adult (20–39 years)	Health education	Complete physical examination at about 20 years, then every 5–6 years
	Weight management with good nutrition as basal metabolic rate changes	Cancer checkup every 3 years
	Life-style counseling	Female: breast self-examination monthly
	Stress management skills	Male: testicular self-examination monthly

Safe driving
Family planning
Parenting skills
Regular exercise
Environmental health choices
Professional dental hygiene every 6–12 months
Immunization
Tetanus at 20 years and every 10 years
Female: rubella, if zero negative for antibodies

All females: baseline mammography between ages 35 and 40
Parents-to-be: high-risk screening for Down syndrome, Tay-Sachs disease
Pregnant female: screen for sexually transmitted disease, rubella titer, Rh factor
Screening and interventions if high risk
Female with previous breast cancer: annual mammography at 35 years and after
Female with mother or sister who has had breast cancer, same as above
Family history of colorectal cancer or high risk: annual stool guaiac, digital rectal examination, and sigmoidoscopy
PPD if exposed to tuberculosis

Middle-aged adult (40–59 years)

Health education: continue with young adult
Midlife changes, male and female counseling
"Empty-nest syndrome"

Complete physical examination every 5–6 years with complete laboratory evaluation (serum/urine tests, x-ray, ECG)
Cancer checkup every year
Female: breast self-examination monthly

(Continued)

Primary and Secondary Prevention for Age-related Conditions *(Continued)*

Developmental Level	Primary Prevention	Secondary Prevention
	Anticipatory guidance for retirement Grandparenting Professional dental hygiene every 6–12 months Immunizations Tetanus every 10 years Pneumococcal / influenza — annual if high risk; *i.e.*, major chronic disease (COPD, CAD)	Male: testicular self-examination monthly All females: annual mammography 50 years and over Schiøtz tonometry (glaucoma) every 3–5 years Pregnant female: perinatal screening by amniocentesis if desired Sigmoidoscopy at 50 and 51, then every 4 years if negative Stool guaiac annually at 50 and thereafter Screening and intervention if high risk Endometrial cancer: have endometrial sampling at menopause Oral cancer: screen more often if substance abuser
Elderly adult (60–74 years)	Health education: continue with previous counseling Home safety Retirement Loss of spouse Special health needs	Complete physical examination every 2 years with laboratory assessments Annual cancer checkup Blood pressure annually Female: breast self-examination monthly

82

Nutritional changes
Changes in hearing or vision
Alterations in bowel or bladder habits
Professional dental/oral hygiene every 6–12 months
Immunizations
  Tetanus every 10 years
  Pneumococcal ⎱ annual if high risk
  influenza ⎰

Male: testicular self-examination monthly
Female: annual mammogram
Annual stool guaiac
Sigmoidoscopy every 4 years
Schiotz tonometry every 3–5 years
Podiatric evaluation with foot care PRN
Screen for high risk
  Depression
  Suicide

Old-age adult (75 years and over)
Health education: continue counsel
Anticipatory guidance
  Dying and death
  Loss of spouse
  Increasing dependency on others
Professional dental/oral hygiene every 6–12 months
Immunizations
  Tetanus every 10 years
  Pneumococcal ⎱ annual
  influenza ⎰

Complete physical examination annually
Laboratory assessments
Cancer checkup
Blood pressure
Stool guaiac
Female: mammogram, sigmoidoscopy every 4 years
Schiotz tonometry every 3–5 years
Podiatrist PRN

Home Maintenance Management, Impaired

DEFINITION

Impaired Home Maintenance Management: The state in which an individual or family experiences or is at risk of experiencing a difficulty in maintaining self or family in a home environment.

Author's Note:

This diagnostic category can describe situations in which the individual and/or family needs specific instruction to manage home care of a family member and/or activities of daily living.

DEFINING CHARACTERISTICS

Major (Must Be Present)

Outward expressions by individual or family of difficulty in maintaining the home (cleaning, repairs, financial needs)
or
In caring for self or family member at home

Minor (May Be Present)

Poor hygienic practices
   Infections   Infestations
   Accumulated wastes

Unwashed cooking
and eating
equipment

Offensive odors

Impaired caregiver
Overtaxed
Anxious

Lack of knowledge
Negative response to
ill member

Unavailable support system

ETIOLOGICAL, CONTRIBUTING, RISK FACTORS

Pathophysiological

Chronic debilitating disease
Diabetes mellitus
Chronic obstructive
pulmonary
disease
Congestive heart
failure
Cancer

Arthritis
Multiple sclerosis
Muscular dystrophy
Parkinsonian
syndrome
Cerebrovascular
accident

Situational (Personal, Environmental)

Injury to individual or family member (fractured
limb, spinal cord injury)
Surgery (amputation, ostomy)
Impaired mental status (memory lapses,
depression, anxiety—severe, panic)
Substance abuse (alcohol, other drugs)
Unavailable support system
Loss of family member
Addition of family member (newborn, aged
parent)
Lack of knowledge
Insufficient finances

Maturational

Infant
Newborn care
High risk for sudden infant death syndrome
(SIDS)
Elderly
Family member with deficits (cognitive,
motor, sensory)

Hopelessness

DEFINITION

Hopelessness: A sustained subjective emotional state in which an individual sees no alternatives or personal choices available to solve problems or to achieve what is desired and cannot mobilize energy on own behalf to establish goals.

Author's Note:

Hopelessness differs from powerlessness in that a hopeless person sees no solution to his problem and/or way to achieve what is desired, even if he/she has control of his/her life. A powerless person may see an alternative or answer to the problem yet be unable to do anything about it because of perceived lack of control and resources.

DEFINING CHARACTERISTICS

Major (Must Be Present)

Expresses profound, overwhelming apathy in response to a situation perceived as impossible with no solutions (overt or covert)

Examples of expressions are

"I might as well give up because I can't make things better."

"My future seems awful to me."

"I can't imagine what my life will be like in ten years."

"I've never been given a break, so why should I in the future?"

"Life looks unpleasant when I think ahead."

"I know I'll never get what I really want."

"Things never work out how I want them to."

"It's foolish to want to get anything because I
    never do."
"It's unlikely that I'll get satisfaction in the
    future."
"The future seems vague and uncertain."

Physiological
  Slowed responses to stimuli

Emotional
  The hopeless person often has difficulty
      experiencing feelings, but may feel
    Unable to seek good fortune, luck, or God's
      favor
    That he/she has no meaning or purpose in life
    "Empty or drained"
    A sense of loss and deprivation

Person exhibits
  Passiveness
  Decreased verbalization
  Lack of ambition, initiative, and interest

Cognitive
  Decreased problem-solving and decision-making
    capabilities
  Deals with past and future, not the here and now
  Decreased flexibility in thought processes
  Lacks imagination and wishing capabilities
  Unable to identify and/or accomplish desired
    objectives and goals
  Unable to plan, organize, or make decisions
  Unable to recognize sources of hope

Minor (May Be Present)

Physiological
  Anorexia
  Weight loss
  Decreased exercise
  Increased sleep

Emotional
  Patient feels
    Incompetent
    "A lump in the throat"
    Discouraged with self and others
    "At the end of his/her rope"
    Tense

Helpless

Overwhelmed ("I just can't . . .")

Loss of gratification from roles and
    relationships

Vulnerable

Person exhibits

Poor eye contact; turns away from speaker;
    shrugs in response to speaker

Apathy (decreased response to internal and
    external stimuli)

Decreased affect

Decreased motivation

Despondency

Sighing

Social withdrawal

Lack of involvement in self-care (may be
    cooperative in nursing care but offers little
    help to self)

Passively *allows* care

Regression

Resignation

Depression

Anger

Destructiveness

Cognitive

Conveys negative and/or slowed thought
    processes

Decreased ability to integrate information
    received

Loss of time perception for past, present, and
    future

Decreased ability to recall from the past

Confusion

Inability to communicate effectively

Distorted thought perceptions and associations

Unreasonable judgment

Suicidal thoughts

Unrealistic perceptions in relation to hope

ETIOLOGICAL, CONTRIBUTING, RISK FACTORS

Pathophysiological

Any chronic and/or terminal illness can cause or
    contribute to hopelessness (heart disease,

kidney disease, cancer, acquired
immunodeficiency syndrome [AIDS]).
Associated factors include
Failing or deteriorating physiological
condition
Impaired body image
New and unexpected signs or symptoms of
previous disease process
Prolonged pain, discomfort, weakness
Impaired functional abilities (walking,
elimination, eating)

Treatment-related

Prolonged treatments (*e.g.,* chemotherapy,
radiation) that cause discomfort
Prolonged treatments with no positive results
Treatments that alter body image (*e.g.,* surgery,
chemotherapy)
Prolonged diagnostic studies with no results
Prolonged dependence on equipment for life
support (dialysis, ventilator)
Prolonged dependence on equipment for
monitoring bodily functions (telemetry)

Situational (Personal, Environmental)

Prolonged activity restriction (*e.g.,* fractures,
spinal cord injury)
Prolonged isolation for disease processes (*e.g.,*
infectious diseases, reverse isolation for
compromised immune system)
Separation from significant others (parents,
spouse, children, others)
Inability to achieve goals that one values in life
(marriage, education, children)
Inability to participate in activities one desires
(walking, sports)
Loss of something or someone valued (spouse,
children, friend, financial resources)
Prolonged caretaking responsibilities (spouse,
child, parent)
Exposure to long-term physiological or
psychological stress
Loss of belief in transcendent values/God

Maturational

Child
  Loss of caregivers
  Loss of trust in significant other (parents, sibling)
  Abandonment by caregivers
  Loss of autonomy related to illness (*e.g.,* fracture)
  Loss of bodily functions
  Inability to achieve developmental tasks (trust, autonomy, initiative, industry)
Adolescent
  Loss of significant other (peer, family)
  Loss of bodily functions
  Change in body image
  Inability to achieve developmental task (role identity)
Adult
  Impaired bodily functions, loss of body part
  Impaired relationships (separation, divorce)
  Loss of job, career
  Loss of significant others (death of children, spouse)
  Inability to achieve developmental tasks (intimacy, commitment, productivity)
Elderly
  Sensory deficits
  Motor deficits
  Loss of independence
  Loss of significant others, things
  Inability to achieve developmental tasks (integrity)

Infection, Potential for

Infection Transmission, Potential for

DEFINITION

Potential for Infection: The state in which an individual is at risk of being invaded by an opportunistic or pathogenic agent (virus, fungus, bacterium, protozoan, or other parasite) from external sources.

> **Author's Note:**
> Potential for Infection describes a situation when host defenses are compromised, making the host more susceptible to environmental pathogens.

DEFINING CHARACTERISTICS

Major (Must Be Present)

Evidence of risk factors, such as
Altered production of leukocytes
Altered immune response
Altered circulation (lymph, blood)
Presence of favorable conditions for infection
(see Etiological, Contributing, Risk
Factors)
History of infection

ETIOLOGICAL, CONTRIBUTING, RISK FACTORS

A variety of health problems and situations can create conditions that would encourage the development of infections. Some common factors are listed below.

Pathophysiological

Chronic diseases
Cancer
Renal failure
Arthritis
Hematologic
disorders
Diabetes mellitus
Hepatic disorders
Respiratory
disorders
Collagen diseases
Heritable disorders

Alcoholism
Immunosuppression
Immunodeficiency
Altered or insufficient leukocytes
Blood dyscrasias
Impaired oxygen transport
Altered integumentary system
Periodontal disease
Obesity
Loss of consciousness
Hormonal factors

Treatment-related

Medications
  Antibiotics
  Corticosteroids
  Antiviral agents
  Insulin
  Antifungal agents
  Tranquilizers
  Immuno-
    suppressants
Surgery
Radiation therapy
Dialysis
Total parenteral
  nutrition
Tracheostomy
Chemotherapy
Lack of
  immunizations
Presence of invasive
  lines (e.g., IVs,
  Foley catheter,
  enteral feedings)

Situational (Personal, Environmental)

Prolonged immobility
Trauma (accidental, intentional)
Postpartum period
Contact with contagious agents (nosocomial or
    community-acquired)
Postoperative period
Increased length of hospital stay
Malnutrition
Stress
Bites (animal, insect, human)
Thermal injuries
Warm, moist, dark environment (skinfolds,
    casts)
Inadequate personal hygiene
Lack of immunizations
Smoking

Maturational

Newborn
  Lack of maternal antibodies (dependent on
      maternal exposure)
  Lack of normal flora
  Open wounds (umbilical, circumcision)
  Immature immune system
Infant/child
  Lack of immunization
Elderly
  Debilitated
  Decreased immune response
  Chronic diseases

Infection Transmission, Potential for*

DEFINITION

Potential for Infection Transmission: The state in
which an individual is at risk for transferring an opportunistic or pathogenic agent to others.

DEFINING CHARACTERISTICS

Major (Must Be Present)

Presence of risk factors (see Etiological,
    Contributing, Risk Factors)

ETIOLOGICAL, CONTRIBUTING, RISK FACTORS

Pathophysiological

Colonization with highly antibiotic-resistant
    organism
Airborne transmission exposure

---

* This diagnostic category is not currently on the NANDA
list but has been included for clarity or usefulness.

Contact transmission exposure (direct, indirect, contact droplet)
Vehicle transmission exposure
Vector-borne transmission exposure

Treatment-related

Contaminated or dirty surgical procedures (incision and drainage, traumatic wound)
Drainage devices (urinary, chest tubes)
Suction equipment
Invasive devices (endotracheal tubes)

Situational (Personal, Environmental)

Disaster with hazardous infectious material
Unsanitary living conditions (sewage, personal hygiene)
Areas considered high risk for vector-borne diseases (malaria, rabies, bubonic plague)
Areas considered high risk for vehicle-borne disease (hepatitis A, shigella, salmonella)
Lack of knowledge
Intravenous drug use
Multiple sexual partners

Maturational

Newborn
Birth outside a hospital setting in an uncontrolled environment
Exposure during prenatal or perinatal period to communicable disease via mother

Injury, Potential for

Aspiration, Potential for

Poisoning, Potential for

Suffocation, Potential for

Trauma, Potential for

DEFINITION

Potential for Injury: The state in which an individual is at risk for harm because of a perceptual or physiological deficit, a lack of awareness of hazards, or maturational age.

> **Author's Note:**
> This diagnostic category has four subcategories: Potential for Aspiration, Poisoning, Suffocation, and Trauma. Should the nurse choose to isolate interventions only for prevention of poisoning, then the diagnostic category Potential for Poisoning would be useful.

DEFINING CHARACTERISTICS

Major (Must Be Present)

Presence of risk factors such as (see Etiological, Contributing, Risk Factors for specific factors)
Evidence of environmental hazards
Lack of knowledge of environmental hazards
Lack of knowledge of safety precautions
History of accidents
Impaired mobility
Sensory deficits

ETIOLOGICAL, CONTRIBUTING, RISK FACTORS

Pathophysiological

Altered cerebral function
Tissue hypoxia   Syncope
Post-trauma   Confusion
Vertigo
Altered mobility
Unsteady gait   Loss of limb

Impaired sensory function
   Vision   Thermal/touch
   Hearing   Smell
Pain
Fatigue
Orthostatic hypotension
Vertebrobasilar insufficiency
Cervical spondylosis
Subclavian steal
Vestibular disorders
Carotid sinus syncope
Seizures
Hypoglycemia
Electrolyte imbalance
Amputation
Arthritis
Cerebrovascular accident
Parkinsonism
Congestive heart failure
Dysrhythmias
Depression

Treatment-related

Medications
   Sedatives   Hypoglycemics
   Vasodilators   Diuretics
   Antihypertensives   Phenothiazines
Casts/crutches, canes, walkers

Situational (Personal, Environmental)

Decrease in or loss of short-term memory
Dehydration (*e.g.,* summer)
Prolonged bed rest
Stress
Vasovagal reflex
Faulty judgment
Alcohol
Poisons (plants, toxic chemicals)
Household hazards
   Unsafe walkways   Faulty electric wires
   Unsafe toys   Improperly stored
                     poisons

Automotive hazards
  Lack of use of seatbelts or child seats   Mechanically unsafe vehicle
Fire hazards
  Smoking in bed   Improperly stored petroleum products
  Gas leaks
Unfamiliar setting (hospital, nursing home)
Improper footwear
Inattentive caretaker
Improper use of aids (crutches, canes, walkers, wheelchairs)
Environmental hazards (home, school, hospital)
History of accidents

Maturational

Infant/child
  High risk for maturational age
    Suffocation hazards (improper crib, pillow in crib, plastic bags, unattended in water—bath, pool, choking on such things as toys or food)
    Improper use of bicycles, kitchen utensils/ appliances, sports equipment, lawn equipment
    Poison (plants, cleaning agents, medications)
    Fire (matches, fireplace, stove)
    Falls
Adolescent
  Automobile
  Bicycle
  Alcohol
  Drugs
Adult
  Drugs
  Automobile
  Alcohol
Elderly
  Motor and sensory deficits
  Medication (accidental overdose, sedation)
  Cognitive deficits

Aspiration, Potential for

DEFINITION

Potential for Aspiration: The state in which an individual is at risk for entry of secretions, solids, or fluids into the tracheobronchial passages.

DEFINING CHARACTERISTICS

Major (Must Be Present)

Presence of risk factors (see Etiological, Contributing, Risk Factors)

ETIOLOGICAL, CONTRIBUTING, RISK FACTORS

Pathophysiological

Reduced level of consciousness
  Anesthesia
  Head injury
  Seizures
  Intoxicated
  Drug overdose
  Cerebrovascular
    accident (CVA)
  Coma
  Presenile dementia
Depressed cough and gag reflexes
Increased intragastric pressure
  Lithotomy position
  Enlarged uterus
  Obesity
  Ascites
Hiatal hernia
Delayed gastric emptying
  Intestinal
    obstruction
  Ileus
  Gastric outlet
    syndrome
Impaired swallowing
  Achalasia
  Scleroderma
  Hiatal hernia
  Esophageal
    strictures
  Myasthenia gravis
  Guillain-Barré
    syndrome
  Multiple sclerosis
  Muscular dystrophy
Impaired ability to chew
Facial/oral/neck surgery or trauma
Paraplegia or hemiplegia

Cerebrovascular accident (CVA)
Parkinsonism
Debilitating conditions
Catatonia
Tracheoesophageal fistula

Treatment-related

Presence of tracheostomy/endotracheal tube
Gastrointestinal tubes
Tube feedings
Medication administration
Wired jaws
Imposed prone position

Situational (Personal, Environmental)

Impaired ability to elevate upper body
Eating when intoxicated

Maturational

Premature
    Impaired sucking/swallowing reflexes
Neonate
    Decreased muscle tone of inferior esophageal
        sphincter
Elderly
    Poor dentition

Poisoning, Potential for

DEFINITION

Potential for Poisoning: The state in which an individual is at high risk of accidental exposure to or ingestion of drugs or dangerous substances.

DEFINING CHARACTERISTICS

Major (Must Be Present)

Presence of risk factors (see Etiological,
    Contributing, Risk Factors under Potential
    for Injury)

Suffocation, Potential for

DEFINITION

Potential for Suffocation: The state in which an individual is at risk for smothering and asphyxiation.

DEFINING CHARACTERISTICS

Major (Must Be Present)

Presence of risk factors (see Etiological, Contributing, Risk Factors under Potential for Injury)

Trauma, Potential for

DEFINITION

Potential for Trauma: The state in which an individual is at high risk of accidental tissue injury (*e.g.,* wound, burns, fracture)

DEFINING CHARACTERISTICS

Major (Must Be Present)

Presence of risk factors (see Etiological, Contributing, Risk Factors under Potential for Injury)

Knowledge Deficit

DEFINITION

Knowledge Deficit: The state in which an individual or group experiences a deficiency in cognitive knowledge or psychomotor skills regarding the condition or treatment plan.

Author's Note:
Knowledge Deficit does not represent a human response, alteration, or pattern of dysfunction but rather an etiological or contributing factor.* Lack of knowledge can contribute to a variety of responses, *e.g.,* anxiety, self-care deficits. All nursing diagnostic categories have related patient/family teaching as a part of nursing interventions, *e.g.,* Altered Bowel Elimination, Impaired Verbal Communication. When the teaching directly relates to a specific nursing diagnosis, incorporate the teaching into the plan. When specific teaching is indicated prior to a procedure, the diagnosis Anxiety related to unfamiliar environment or procedure can be used. When information-giving is directed to assist a person or family with a decision, the diagnosis Decisional Conflict may be indicated.

DEFINING CHARACTERISTICS

Major (Must Be Present)

Verbalizes a deficiency in knowledge or skill/ request for information
Expresses an inaccurate perception of health status
Does not correctly perform a desired or prescribed health behavior

Minor (May Be Present)

Lack of integration of treatment plan into daily activities
Exhibits or expresses psychological alteration (*e.g.,* anxiety, depression) resulting from misinformation or lack of information

* Jenny J: Knowledge Deficit: Not a Nursing Diagnosis. Image 19(4): 184–185, 1987

Mobility, Impaired Physical

DEFINITION

Impaired Physical Mobility: The state in which an individual experiences or is at risk of experiencing limitation of purposeful/independent physical movement.

> **Author's Note:**
> This diagnostic category describes an individual with limited use of arm(s) or leg(s). Nursing interventions would focus on strengthening and restoring function and preventing deterioration. Frequently, the impaired mobility becomes the etiology for other nursing diagnoses such as Self-care Deficit. Potential for Injury, and Potential for Disuse Syndrome.

DEFINING CHARACTERISTICS

Major (Must Be Present)

Inability to move purposefully within the environment, including bed mobility, transfers, ambulation

Minor (May Be Present)

Range-of-motion limitations
Limited muscle strength or control
Impaired coordination

ETIOLOGICAL, CONTRIBUTING, RISK FACTORS

Pathophysiological

Neuromuscular impairment
Autoimmune alterations (multiple sclerosis, arthritis)

Nervous system diseases (parkinsonism,
    myasthenia gravis)
Muscular dystrophy
Partial or total paralysis (spinal cord injury,
    stroke)
Central nervous system (CNS) tumor
Increased intracranial pressure
Sensory deficits
Musculoskeletal impairment
    Spasms
    Flaccidity, atrophy, weakness
    Connective-tissue disease (systemic lupus
        erythematosus)
    Edema (increased synovial fluid)

Treatment-related

External devices (casts or splints, braces, IV
    tubing)
Surgical procedures (amputation)

Situational (Personal, Environmental)

Trauma or surgical procedures
Nonfunctioning or missing limbs (fractures)
Pain

Maturational

Elderly
    Decreased motor agility
    Muscle weakness

Noncompliance

DEFINITION

Noncompliance: The state in which an individual or group desires to comply, but factors are present that deter adherence to health-related advice given by health professionals.

DEFINING CHARACTERISTICS

Major (Must Be Present)

Verbalization of noncompliance or
nonparticipation or confusion about therapy
and/or
Direct observation of behavior indicating
noncompliance

Minor (May Be Present)

Missed appointments
Partially used or unused medications
Persistence of symptoms
Progression of disease process
Occurrence of undesired outcomes
(postoperative morbidity, pregnancy,
obesity, addiction, regression during
rehabilitation)

ETIOLOGICAL, CONTRIBUTING, RISK FACTORS

Pathophysiological

Impaired ability to perform tasks because of
disability (*e.g.,* poor memory, motor and
sensory deficits)
Chronic nature of illness
Increasing amount of disease-related symptoms
despite adherence to advised regimen

Treatment-related

Side-effects of therapy
Previous unsuccessful experiences with advised regimen
Impersonal aspects of referral process
Nontherapeutic environment
Complex, unsupervised, or prolonged therapy
Financial cost of therapy
Nontherapeutic relationship between client and nurse

Situational (Personal, Environmental)

Concurrent illness of family member
Inclement weather keeping client from keeping appointment
Nonsupportive family, peers, community
Knowledge deficit
Lack of autonomy in health-seeking behavior
Health beliefs run counter to professional advice
Poor self-esteem
Disturbance in body image

Maturational

Developmental maturity of the client is incompatible with his/her age.

Nutrition, Altered: Less Than Body Requirements

Impaired Swallowing

DEFINITION

Altered Nutrition: Less Than Body Requirements: The state in which an individual who is not NPO experiences or is at risk of experiencing reduced weight related to inadequate intake or metabolism of nutrients.

Author's Note:

This diagnostic category describes individuals who can ingest food but only in less-than-adequate amounts. This category should not be used to describe individuals who are NPO or cannot ingest food. These situations should be described by the collaborative problem of

Potential Complication:
Electrolyte imbalances
Negative nitrogen balance

Nurses monitor to detect complications of an NPO state and confer with physicians for parenteral therapy. Some nursing diagnoses that may relate to an individual who is NPO are Potential Altered Oral Mucous Membrane and Altered Comfort.

DEFINING CHARACTERISTICS

Major (Must Be Present)

Reported inadequate food intake less than recommended daily allowance (RDA) with or without weight loss
and/or
Actual or potential metabolic needs in excess of intake

Minor (May Be Present)

Weight 10% to 20% or more below ideal for height and frame
Triceps skin fold, mid-arm circumference, and mid-arm muscle circumference less than 60% standard measurement
Tachycardia on minimal exercise and bradycardia at rest
Muscle weakness and tenderness
Mental irritability or confusion
Decreased serum albumin

Decreased serum transferrin or iron-binding
      capacity
Decreased lymphocyte count

ETIOLOGICAL, CONTRIBUTING, RISK FACTORS

Pathophysiological

Hyperanabolic/catabolic states
  Burns (postacute   Cancer
        phase)   Trauma
  Infection
Chemical dependence
Faulty metabolism
  Cirrhosis
  Gastric resection
Dysphagia
  Cerebrovascular   Parkinson's disease
        accident   Neuromuscular
  Amyotrophic lateral   disorders
        sclerosis   Muscular dystrophy
  Cerebral palsy
Absorptive disorders
  Crohn's disease
  Cystic fibrosis
Diverticulosis
Stomatitis
Trauma
Altered level of consciousness
Fear of choking

Treatment-related

Surgery
Medications (cancer chemotherapy)
Surgical reconstruction of the mouth
Wired jaw
Radiation therapy
Inadequate absorption as a side-effect
  Colchicine
  Pyrimethamine
  Antacid
  Neomycin
  Para-aminosalicylic acid

Situational (Personal, Environmental)

Anorexia
Depression
Stress
Social isolation
Nausea and vomiting
Allergies
Parasites
Inability to procure food (physical limitations,
    financial or transportation problems)
Lack of knowledge of adequate nutrition
Crash or fad diet
Inability to chew (wired jaw, damaged or missing
    teeth, ill-fitting dentures)
Diarrhea
Lactose intolerance
Ethnic/religious eating patterns

Maturational

Infant/child
    Congenital anomalies
    Growth spurts
    Developmental eating disorders
Adolescent
    Anorexia nervosa (postacute phase)
Elderly
    Altered sense of taste

Impaired Swallowing

DEFINITION

Impaired Swallowing: The state in which an individual has decreased ability to voluntarily pass fluids and/or solid foods from the mouth to the stomach.

DEFINING CHARACTERISTICS

Major (Must Be Present)

Observed evidence of difficulty in swallowing
and/or
Stasis of food in oral cavity
Evidence of aspiration

Minor (May Be Present)

Coughing
Choking
Apraxia (ideational, constructional, or visual)

ETIOLOGICAL, CONTRIBUTING, RISK FACTORS

Pathophysiological

Cleft lip/palate
Neuromuscular disorders (*e.g.,* cerebral palsy,
    muscular dystrophy, amyotrophic lateral
    sclerosis, myasthenia gravis, Guillain-Barré
    syndrome, botulism, poliomyelitis,
    parkinsonism)
Neoplastic disease (disease affecting brain and/or
    brain stem)
Cerebrovascular accident
Right or left hemispheric damage to the brain
Damage to the 5th, 7th, 9th, 10th, or 11th
    cranial nerves
Tracheoesophageal fistula
Tracheoesophageal tumors, edema

Treatment-related

Surgical reconstruction of the mouth and/or
    throat
Anesthesia
Mechanical obstruction (tracheostomy tube)

Situational (Personal, Environmental)

Altered level of consciousness
Fatigue
Limited awareness
Altered sense of taste
Irritated oropharyngeal cavity

Maturational

Infant/child
    Congenital anomalies
    Developmental disorders

Nutrition, Altered: More Than Body Requirements

DEFINITION

Altered Nutrition: More Than Body Requirements: The state in which an individual experiences or is at risk of experiencing weight gain related to an intake in excess of metabolic requirements.

Author's Note:

Obesity is a complex condition with sociocultural, psychological, and metabolic implications. This diagnostic category, when used to describe obesity or overweight conditions, focuses on them as nutritional problems. The focus of treatment is behavioral modification and life-style changes. It is recommended that Altered Health Maintenance related to intake in excess of metabolic requirements be used in place of this diagnostic category. When weight gain is the result of physiological conditions, *e.g.,* altered taste or pharmacological interventions such as corticosteroid therapy, this diagnostic category can be clinically useful.

DEFINING CHARACTERISTICS

Major (Must Be Present)

Overweight (weight 10% over ideal for height and frame)

or

Obese (weight 20% or more over ideal for height and frame)

Triceps skin fold greater than 15 mm in men and 25 mm in women

Minor (May Be Present)

Reported undesirable eating patterns
Intake in excess of metabolic requirements
Sedentary activity patterns

ETIOLOGICAL, CONTRIBUTING, RISK FACTORS
Pathophysiological

Altered satiety patterns
Decreased sense of taste and smell

Treatment-related

Medications (corticosteroids)
Radiation (decreased sense of taste and smell)

Situational (Personal, Environmental)

Pregnancy (at risk to gain more than 25–30 pounds)
Lack of basic nutritional knowledge

Maturational

Adult/elderly
Decreased activity patterns
Decreased metabolic needs

Nutrition, Altered: Potential for More Than Body Requirements

DEFINITION

Altered Nutrition: Potential for More Than Body Requirements: The state in which an individual is at risk of experiencing an intake of nutrients that exceeds metabolic needs.

> **Author's Note:**
> This diagnostic category is similar to Potential Altered Nutrition: More Than Body Requirements. It describes an individual who has a family history of obesity, who is demonstrating a pattern of higher weight, and/or who has had a history of excessive weight gain (*e.g.,* previous pregnancy). Until clinical research differentiates this category from other presently accepted categories, use Altered Health Maintenance (Actual or Potential) or Potential Altered Nutrition: More Than Body Requirements to direct teaching to assist families and individuals to identify unhealthy dietary patterns.

DEFINING CHARACTERISTICS

Reported or observed obesity in one or both parents

Rapid transition across growth percentiles in infants or children

Reported use of solid food as major food source before 5 months of age

Observed use of food as a reward or comfort measure

Reported or observed higher baseline weight at beginning of each pregnancy

Dysfunctional eating patterns

Parenting, Altered

Parental Role Conflict

DEFINITION

Altered Parenting: The state in which one or more caregivers experience a real or potential inability to provide a constructive environment that nurtures the growth and development of his/her/their child (children).

Author's Note:
A family's ability to function is at a high risk of developing problems when the child or parent has a condition that increases the stress of the family unit. The term *parent* refers to any individual(s) defined as the primary caregiver(s) for a child.

DEFINING CHARACTERISTICS

Major (Must Be Present)

Inappropriate parenting behaviors and/or lack of parental attachment behavior

Minor (May Be Present)

Frequent verbalization of dissatisfaction or disappointment with infant/child
Verbalization of frustration of role
Verbalization of perceived or actual inadequacy
Diminished or inappropriate visual, tactile, or auditory stimulation of infant
Evidence of abuse or neglect of child
Growth and development lag in infant/child

ETIOLOGICAL, CONTRIBUTING, RISK FACTORS

Individuals or families who may be at high risk for developing or experiencing parenting difficulties
Parent(s)
Single
Adolescent
Abusive
Emotionally disturbed
Alcoholic
Addicted to drugs
Terminally ill
Acutely disabled
Accident victim
Child
Of unwanted pregnancy
Of undesired gender
Physically handicapped
Mentally handicapped

With undesired	Hyperactive
characteristics	Terminally ill
	Rebellious

Situational (Personal, Environmental)

Separation from nuclear family
Lack of extended family
Lack of knowledge
Economic problems
   Inflation   Unemployment
Relationship problems
   Marital discord   Live-in sexual
   Divorce   partner
   Separation   Relocation
   Step-parents
Change in family unit
   New child   Relative moves in

Other

History of ineffective relationships with own
    parents
Parental history of abusive relationship with
    parents
Unrealistic expectations of child by parent
Unrealistic expectations of self by parent
Unrealistic expectations of parent by child
Unmet psychosocial needs of child by parent
Unmet psychosocial needs of parent by child

Parental Role Conflict

DEFINITION

Parental Role Conflict: The state in which a parent
experiences or perceives a change in role in response
to external factors (*e.g.,* illness, hospitalization, divorce, separation).

Author's Note:
This diagnostic category describes a parent or parents
whose previously effective functioning ability is
(Continued)

Author's Note (Continued)

challenged by external factors. In certain situations, such as illness, role confusion and conflict are expected. This category differs from Altered Parenting, which describes a parent or parents that demonstrate or are at high risk of demonstrating inappropriate parenting behaviors and/or lack of parental attachment. If parents are not assisted in adapting their role to external factors, Parental Role Conflict can lead to Altered Parenting. The term *parent* refers to any individual(s) defined as the primary caregiver(s) for a child.

This diagnostic category was developed by the Nursing Diagnosis Discussion Group, Rainbow Babies' and Children's Hospital, University Hospitals of Cleveland.

DEFINING CHARACTERISTICS

Major (Must Be Present)

Parent(s) express concerns about changes in parental role
and/or
Demonstrated disruption in care-giving routines

Minor (May Be Present)

Parent(s) expresses concerns/feelings of inadequacy to provide for child's physical and emotional needs during hospitalization or in the home.

Parent(s) expresses concern about effect of child's illness on family

Parent(s) expresses concerns about care of siblings at home

Parent(s) expresses guilt about contributing to the child's illness through lack of knowledge, judgment, and so forth

Parent(s) expresses concern about perceived loss of control over decisions relating to the child

Parent(s) reluctant, unable, or unwilling to participate in normal caregiving activities even with encouragement and support

Parent(s) verbalizes/demonstrates feelings of guilt, anger, fear, anxiety, and/or frustration

ETIOLOGICAL, CONTRIBUTING, RISK FACTORS

Situational (Personal, Environmental)

Illness of child
  Birth of a child with a congenital defect and/
    or chronic illness
  Hospitalization of a child with an acute or
    chronic illness
  Change in acuity, prognosis, or environment
    of care (*e.g.,* transfer to or from an ICU)
  Invasive or restrictive treatment modalities
    (*e.g.,* isolation, intubation)
  Home care of a child with special needs (*e.g.,*
    apnea monitoring, postural drainage,
    hyperalimentation)
  Interruptions of family life due to treatment
    regimen
Separation
  Divorce
  Remarriage
  Death
  Illness of caregiver
Change in family membership
  Birth, adoption
  Addition of relatives (*e.g.,* grandparent,
    siblings)

Post-trauma Response

Rape Trauma Syndrome

DEFINITION

Post-trauma Response: The state in which an individual experiences a sustained painful response to (an) overwhelming traumatic event(s) that has (have) not been assimilated.

DEFINING CHARACTERISTICS

Major (Must Be Present)

Reexperience of the traumatic event, which may be identified in cognitive, affective, and/or sensory-motor activities such as

Flashbacks, intrusive thoughts

Repetitive dreams/nightmares

Excessive verbalization of the traumatic events

Survival guilt or guilt about behavior required for survival

Painful emotion, self-blame, shame, or sadness

Vulnerability or helplessness, anxiety, or panic

Fear of

Repetition

Death

Loss of bodily control

Anger outburst/rage, startle reaction

Hyperalertness or hypervigilance

Minor (May Be Present)

Psychic/emotional numbness

Impaired interpretation of reality, impaired memory

Confusion, dissociation, or amnesia

Vagueness about traumatic event

Narrowed attention, or inattention/daze

Feeling of numbness, constricted affect

Feeling detached/alienated

Reduced interest in significant activities

Rigid role-adherence or stereotyped behavior

Altered life-style

Submissiveness, passiveness, or dependency

Self-destructiveness (alcohol/drug abuse, suicide attempts, reckless driving, illegal activities, etc.)

Difficulty with interpersonal relationships

Development of phobia regarding trauma

Avoidance of situations or activities that arouse recollection of the trauma

Social isolation/withdrawal, negative self-concept

Sleep disturbances, emotional disturbances

Irritability, poor impulse control, or explosiveness

Loss of faith in people or the world/feeling of
meaninglessness in life
Chronic anxiety or/and chronic depression
Somatic preoccupation/multiple physiological
symptoms

ETIOLOGICAL, CONTRIBUTING, RISK FACTORS

Situational (Personal, Environmental)

Traumatic events of natural origin, including
Floods
Earthquakes
Volcanic eruptions
Storms
Avalanches
Epidemics (may be of human origin)
Other natural disasters, which are
overwhelming to most people
Traumatic events of human origin, such as
Wars
Airplane crashes
Serious car accidents
Large fires
Bombing
Concentration camp confinement
Torture
Assault
Rape
Industrial disasters (nuclear, chemical, or
other life-threatening accidents)
Other traumatic events of human origin that
involve death and destruction or the
threat of them

Rape Trauma Syndrome

DEFINITION

Rape Trauma Syndrome: The state in which an individual experiences a forced, violent sexual assault (vaginal or anal penetration) against his or her will and without his or her consent. The trauma syndrome that develops from this attack or attempted attack includes an acute phase of disorganization of the victim and family's life-style and a long-term process of reorganization of life-style.*

DEFINING CHARACTERISTICS

Major (Must Be Present)

Reports or evidence of sexual assault

Minor (May Be Present)

If the victim is a child, parent(s) may experience similar responses.

Acute phase
Somatic responses
    Gastrointestinal irritability (nausea, vomiting, anorexia)
    Genitourinary discomfort (pain, pruritus)
    Skeletal muscle tension (spasms, pain)
Psychological responses
    Denial
    Emotional shock
    Anger
    Fear—of being alone or that the rapist will return (a child victim will fear punishment, repercussions, abandonment, rejection)
    Guilt
    Panic on seeing assailant or scene of attack
Sexual responses
    Mistrust of men (if victim is a woman)
    Change in sexual behavior
Long-term phase

Any response of the acute phase may continue if resolution does not occur.

Psychological responses
    Phobias
    Nightmares or sleep disturbances

* Holmstrom L, Burgess AW: Development of diagnostic categories: Sexual traumas. Am J Nurs 75:1288–1291, 1975

Anxiety
Depression

Powerlessness

DEFINITION

Powerlessness: The state in which an individual or group perceives a lack of personal control over certain events or situations.

> **Author's Note:**
> Most individuals are subject to feelings of powerlessness in varying degrees in various situations. This diagnostic category can be used to describe individuals who respond to loss of control with apathy, anger, or depression. Pronged states of powerlessness may lead to hopelessness.

DEFINING CHARACTERISTICS

Major (Must Be Present)

Overt or covert expressions of dissatisfaction over inability to control situation (*e.g.,* illness, prognosis, care, recovery rate)

Minor (May Be Present)

Refuses or is reluctant to participate in decision-making

Apathy	Uneasiness
Aggressive behavior	Resignation
Violent behavior	Acting-out behavior
Anxiety	Depression

ETIOLOGICAL, CONTRIBUTING, RISK FACTORS

Pathophysiological

Any disease process—acute or chronic—can contribute to powerlessness. Some common sources are the following:

Inability to communicate (CVA, Guillain-Barré syndrome, intubation)

Inability to perform activities of daily living (CVA, cervical trauma, myocardial infarction, pain)

Inability to perform role responsibilities (surgery, trauma, arthritis)

Progressive debilitating disease (multiple sclerosis, terminal cancer)

Mental illness

Substance abuse

Obesity

Disfigurement

Situational (Personal, Environmental)

Lack of knowledge

Personal characteristics that highly value control (*e.g.,* internal locus of control)

Hospital or institutional limitations

Some control relinquished to others	Lack of consultation regarding decisions
No privacy	Social displacement
Altered personal territory	Relocation
Social isolation	Insufficient finances
Lack of explanations from caregivers	Sexual harassment

Maturational

Adolescent
Dependence on peer group
Independence from family
Young adult
Marriage

Pregnancy
Parenthood
Adult
    Adolescent children
    Physical signs of aging
    Career pressures
    Divorce
Elderly
    Sensory deficits
    Motor deficits
    Losses (money, significant others)

Respiratory Function, Potential Altered*

Ineffective Airway Clearance

Ineffective Breathing Patterns

Impaired Gas Exchange

DEFINITION

Potential Altered Respiratory Function (ARF): The state in which an individual is at risk of experiencing a threat to the passage of air through the respiratory tract and to the exchange of gases (O_2–CO_2) between the lungs and the vascular system.

* This diagnostic category is not currently on the NANDA list but has been included for clarity or usefulness.

Author's Note:

This diagnostic category has been added by the author to describe a state in which the entire respiratory system may be affected, not just isolated areas such as airway clearance of gas exchange. Smoking, allergy, and immobility are examples of factors that affect the entire system and thus make it incorrect to use Impaired Gas Exchange related to immobility, since immobility also affects airway clearance and breathing patterns. It is advised that Potential Altered Respiratory Function not be used to describe an actual problem, which is a collaborative problem—not a nursing diagnosis. The diagnoses Ineffective Airway Clearance and Ineffective Breathing Patterns can be used when the nurse can definitively alter the contributing factors that are influencing respiratory function; for example, ineffective cough, immobility, or stress. The nurse is cautioned not to use this diagnostic category to describe acute respiratory disorders, which are the primary responsibility of physicians and nurses together (*i.e.,* a collaborative problem). This can be labeled Potential Complication: Acute hypoxia or Potential Complication: Pulmonary edema. When an individual's immobility threatens multiple systems—integumentary, musculoskeletal, vascular, and respiratory—the nurse should use Potential For Disuse Syndrome to describe the entire situation.

DEFINING CHARACTERISTICS

Major (Must Be Present)

Presence of risk factors that can change respiratory function (see Etiological, Contributing, Risk Factors)

ETIOLOGICAL, CONTRIBUTING, RISK FACTORS

The codes IAC (Ineffective Airway Clearance), and IBP (Ineffective Breathing Patterns) are used to indicate factors specific to that diagnosis. Factors without a code relate to all diagnostic categories.

Pathophysiological

Excessive or thick secretions (IAC)
Infection (IAC)
Neuromuscular impairment (ineffective cough)

Diseases of the	Central nervous
nervous system	system (CNS)
(*e.g.,* Guillain-	depression
Barré	Cerebrovascular
syndrome,	accident (CVA,
multiple	stroke)
sclerosis,	
myasthenia	
gravis)	

Allergic response
Hypertrophy or edema of the upper airway
structures—tonsils, adenoids, sinuses (IAC)

Treatment-related

Medications (narcotics, sedatives, analgesics)
Anesthesia, general or spinal (IAC, IBP)
Suppressed cough reflex (IAC)
Decreased oxygen in the inspired air
Bed rest or immobility

Situational (Personal, Environmental)

Surgery or trauma
Pain, fear, anxiety
Fatigue
Mechanical obstruction (IAC)
Improper positioning (IAC)
Altered anatomic structure (IAC)
Tracheostomy
Aspiration
Extreme high or low humidity (IAC)
Smoking
Mouth breathing (IAC, IBP)
Perception/cognitive impairment (IAC)
Severe nonrelieved cough (IAC, IBP)
Exercise intolerance

Maturational

Neonate
Complicated delivery

Prematurity
Cesarean birth
Low birthweight
Infant/child
Asthma or allergies
Increased emesis (potential for aspiration)
Croup
Cystic fibrosis
Small airway
Elderly
Decreased surfactant in the lungs
Decreased elasticity of the lungs
Immobility
Slowing of reflexes

Ineffective Airway Clearance

DEFINITION

Ineffective Airway Clearance: The state in which an individual experiences a real or potential threat to respiratory status related to inability to cough effectively.

DEFINING CHARACTERISTICS

Major (Must Be Present)

Ineffective cough
or
Inability to remove airway secretions

Minor (May Be Present)

Abnormal breath sounds
Abnormal respiratory rate, rhythm, depth

ETIOLOGICAL, CONTRIBUTING, RISK FACTORS

See *Potential Altered Respiratory Function.*

Ineffective Breathing Patterns

DEFINITION

Ineffective Breathing Patterns: The state in which an individual experiences an actual or potential loss of adequate ventilation related to an altered breathing pattern.

Author's Note:

This diagnostic category has little clinical utility except to describe situations that nurses definitively treat, such as hyperventilation. Individuals with periodic apnea and hypoventilation have a collaborative problem that can be labeled: Potential Complication: Respiratory to indicate that the person is to be monitored for a variety of respiratory dysfunctions. If the person is more vulnerable to a specific respiratory complication, the collaborative problem can then be written as Potential Complication: Pneumonia or Potential Complication: Pulmonary embolism. Hyperventilation is a manifestation of anxiety and/or fear. The nurse can use Anxiety or Fear related to (specify event) as manifested by hyperventilation as a more descriptive diagnosis.

DEFINING CHARACTERISTICS

See also Altered Respiratory Function.

Major (Must Be Present)

Changes in respiratory rate or pattern (from baseline)
Changes in pulse (rate, rhythm, quality)

Minor (May Be Present)

Orthopnea
Tachypnea, hyperpnea, hyperventilation
Dysrhythmic respirations
Splinted/guarded respirations

ETIOLOGICAL, CONTRIBUTING, RISK FACTORS

See Potential Altered Respiratory Function.

Impaired Gas Exchange

DEFINITION

Impaired Gas Exchange: The state in which an individual experiences an actual (or may experience a potential) decreased passage of gases (oxygen and carbon dioxide) between the alveoli of the lungs and the vascular system.

Author's Note:

This diagnostic category does not represent a situation for which nurses prescribe definitive treatment. Nurses do not treat impaired gs exchange, but nurses can treat the functional health patterns that decreased oxygenation can affect, such as activity, sleep, nutrition, and sexual function. Thus, Activity Intolerance related to insufficient oxygenation for ADL better describes the nursing focus. If an individual is at risk or has experienced respiratory dysfunction, the nurse can describe the situation as Potential Complication: Respiratory, or even more specific with Potential Complication: Emboli.

DEFINING CHARACTERISTICS

See also Potential Altered Respiratory Function.

Major (Must Be Present)

Dyspnea on exertion

Minor (May Be Present)

Tendency to assume a three-point position
(sitting, one hand on each knee, bending
forward)

Pursed-lip breathing with prolonged expiratory phase

Increased anteroposterior chest diameter, if chronic

Lethargy and fatigue

Increased pulmonary vascular resistance (increased pulmonary artery/right ventricular pressure)

Decreased gastric motility, prolonged gastric emptying

Decreased oxygen content, decreased oxygen saturation, increased PCO_2, as measured by blood gas studies

Cyanosis

ETIOLOGICAL, CONTRIBUTING, RISK FACTORS

See Potential Altered Respiratory Function.

Role Performance, Altered

DEFINITION

Altered Role Performance: The state in which an individual experiences or is at risk of experiencing a disruption in the way he perceives his role performance.

Author's Note:

This diagnostic category had previously been a subcategory under Self-concept Disturbance. The use of this category in its present state may prove problematic. If a woman was unable to continue her household responsibilities because of illness and these responsibilities were assumed by other family members, the situations that may arise would better be described as Potential Self-concept Disturbance related to re-
(*Continued*)

Author's Note (Continued)
cent loss of role responsibility secondary to illness and Potential Impaired Home Maintenance Management related to lack of knowledge of family members. Until clinical research defines this category more definitively, use Altered Role Performance as a cause of Self-concept Disturbance or Potential Impaired Home Maintenance Management. Should the role disturbance relate to parenting, Parental Role Conflict should be considered.

DEFINING CHARACTERISTICS

Major (Must Be Present)

Conflict related to role perception or performance

Minor (May Be Present)

Change in self-perception of role
Denial of role
Change in others' perception of role
Change in physical capacity to resume role
Lack of knowledge of role
Change in usual patterns of responsibility

Self-care Deficit: (Specify)

DEFINITION

Self-care Deficit: The state in which an individual experiences an impaired motor function or cognitive function, causing a decreased ability to feed, bathe, dress, and/or toilet himself.

DEFINING CHARACTERISTICS

Major (Must Be Present)

Self-feeding deficits
Is unable to open food containers

Is unable to cut food
Is unable to bring food to mouth
Self-bathing deficits (includes washing entire
body, combing hair, brushing teeth,
attending to skin and nail care, and
applying makeup)

Is unable or
unwilling to
wash body or
body parts
Is unable to obtain
water

Is unable to regulate
temperature or
water flow

Self-dressing deficits (including donning regular
or special clothing—not nightclothes)

Has impaired ability
to put on or
take off
clothing
Is unable to fasten
clothing

Is unable to groom
self
satisfactorily
Is unable to obtain
or replace
articles of
clothing

Self-toileting deficits

Is unable or
unwilling to get
to toilet or
commode
Is unable or
unwilling to
carry out
proper hygiene
Is unable to transfer
to and from
toilet or
commode

Is unable to handle
clothing to
accommodate
toileting
Is unable to flush
toilet or empty
commode

Total
Is unable to perform any self-care activities

ETIOLOGICAL, CONTRIBUTING, RISK FACTORS

Pathophysiological

Neuromuscular impairment
Autoimmune alterations (arthritis, multiple
sclerosis)

Metabolic and endocrine alterations (diabetes
mellitus, hypothyroidism)
Nervous system disorders (parkinsonism,
myasthenia gravis, muscular dystrophy,
Guillain-Barré syndrome)
Lack of coordination
Spasticity or flaccidity
Muscular weakness
Partial or total paralysis (spinal cord injury,
stroke)
Central nervous system (CNS) tumors
Increased intracranial pressure
Musculoskeletal disorders
Atrophy
Muscle contractures
Connective tissue diseases (systemic lupus
erythematosus)
Edema (increased synovial fluid)
Visual disorders
Glaucoma
Cataracts
Diabetic/hypertensive retinopathy
Ocular histoplasmosis
Cranial nerve neuropathy
Visual field deficits

Treatment-related

External devices (casts, splints, braces,
intravenous equipment)
Surgical procedures
Fractures   Jejunostomy
Tracheostomy   Ileostomy
Gastrostomy   Colostomy

Situational (Personal, Environmental)

Immobility
Trauma
Nonfunctioning or missing limbs
Coma

Maturational

Elderly
Decreased visual and motor ability
Muscle weakness

Self-concept Disturbance*

Body Image Disturbance

Personal Identity Disturbance

Self-esteem Disturbance

Chronic Low Self-esteem

Situational Low Self-esteem

DEFINITION

Self-concept Disturbance: The state in which an individual experiences or is at risk of experiencing a negative state of change about the way he feels, thinks, or views himself. It may include a change in body image, self-esteem, role performance, or personal identity.

Author's Note:

Self-concept Disturbance represents a broad category under which more specific categories fall. Initially the nurse may not have sufficient clinical data to validate a more specific category as Chronic Low Self-esteem or Body Image Disturbance; thus, Self-concept Disturbance can be used until more specific categories can be supported with data.

---

* This diagnostic category is not currently on the NANDA list but has been included for clarity or usefulness.

DEFINING CHARACTERISTICS

Since a self-concept disturbance may include a change in any one or a combination of its four component parts (body image, self-esteem, role performance, personal identity), and since the nature of the change causing the alteration can be so varied, there is no "typical" response. Reactions may include the following:

Refusal to touch or look at a body part
Refusal to look into a mirror
Unwillingness to discuss a limitation, deformity, or disfigurement
Refusal to accept rehabilitation efforts
Inappropriate attempts to direct own treatment
Denial of the existence of a deformity or disfigurement
Increasing dependence on others
Signs of grieving
   Weeping
   Despair
   Anger
Refusal to participate in own care or take responsibility for self-care (self-neglect)
Self-destructive behavior (alcohol, drug abuse)
Displaying hostility toward the healthy
Withdrawal from social contacts
Changing usual patterns of responsibility
Showing change in ability to estimate relationship of body to environment

ETIOLOGICAL, CONTRIBUTING, RISK FACTORS

A self-concept disturbance can occur as a response to a variety of health problems, situations, and conflicts. Some common sources include the following:

Pathophysiological

Loss of body part(s)
Loss of body function(s)
Severe trauma
Chronic disease

Treatment-related

Hospitalization: chronic or terminal illness
Surgery

Situational (Personal, Environmental)

Divorce, separation from or death of a
significant other
Loss of job or ability to work
Pain
Obesity
Pregnancy
Immobility or loss of function
Need for placement in a nursing home

Maturational

Infant and preschool
Deprivation
Young adult
Peer pressure
Puberty
Middle-aged
Signs of aging (graying or loss of hair)
Reduced hormonal levels (menopause)
Elderly
Losses (people, function, financial, retirement)

Other

Women's movement
Sexual revolution

Body Image Disturbance

DEFINITION

Body Image Disturbance: The state in which an individual experiences or is at risk of experiencing a disruption in the way one perceives one's body image.

DEFINING CHARACTERISTICS

Major (Must Be Present)

Verbal or nonverbal negative response to actual
or perceived change in structure and/or
function

Minor (May Be Present)

Not looking at body part
Not touching body part
Hiding or overexposing body part
Change in social involvement
Negative feelings about body feelings of
    helplessness, hopelessness, powerlessness
Preoccupation with change or loss
Refusal to verify actual change
Depersonalization of part or loss

ETIOLOGICAL, CONTRIBUTING, RISK FACTORS

Pathophysiological

Chronic disease
Loss of body part
Loss of body function
Severe trauma

Treatment-related

Hospitalization
Surgery
Chemotherapy
Radiation

Situational

Pain
Obesity
Pregnancy
Infertility
Immobility
Cultural influences

Maturational

Adolescent
  Puberty
Middle age
  Signs of aging (graying, menopause)
Elderly
  Loss of function

Personal Identity Disturbance

DEFINITION

Personal Identity Disturbance: The state in which an individual experiences or is at risk of experiencing an inability to distinguish between self and nonself.

Author's Note:

This diagnostic category is a subcategory under Self-concept Disturbance. Until clinical research defines and differentiates this category from others, refer to Self-concept Disturbance or Altered Growth and Development for assessment criteria and interventions.

DEFINING CHARACTERISTICS

See Defining Characteristics for Self-concept Disturbance or Altered Growth and Development.

Self-esteem Disturbance

DEFINITION

Self-esteem Disturbance: The state in which an individual experiences or is at risk of experiencing negative self-evaluation about self or capabilities.

Author's Note:

Self-esteem is one of the four components of Self-concept. Self-esteem Disturbance is the general di-
(Continued)

Author's Note (Continued)
agnostic category. Chronic Low Self-esteem and Situational Low Self-esteem represent specific types of Self-esteem Disturbances, thus involving more specific interventions. Initially the nurse may not have sufficient clinical data to validate a more specific diagnosis such as Chronic Low Self-esteem or Situational Low Self-esteem. Refer to the major defining characteristics under these categories for validation.

DEFINING CHARACTERISTICS*

Overt or covert:
Self-negating verbalization
Expressions of shame or guilt
Evaluates self as unable to deal with events
Rationalizes away/rejects positive feedback
and exaggerates negative feedback about
self
Hesitant to try new things/situations
Denial of problems obvious to others
Projection of blame/responsibility for
problems
Rationalizes personal failures
Hypersensitivity to slight criticism
Grandiosity

ETIOLOGICAL, CONTRIBUTING, RISK FACTORS

Self-esteem Disturbance can be either an episodic event or a chronic problem. Failure to resolve a problem or multiple sequential stresses can result in chronic low self-esteem. Those factors that occur over time and are associated with chronic low self-esteem are indicated by chronic low self-esteem.

* Norris J, Kunes-Connell M: Self esteem disturbance: A clinical validation study. In McLane A (ed): Classification of Nursing Diagnoses: Proceedings of the Seventh Conference. St Louis, CV Mosby, 1987

Pathophysiological

Loss of body part(s)
Loss of body function(s)
Disfigurement (trauma, surgery, birth defects)

Situational (Personal, Environmental)

Hospitalization
Loss of job or ability to work
Death of significant other
Separation from significant other
Increase/decrease in weight
Pregnancy
Unemployment
Financial problems
Relationship problems
  Marital discord
  Separation
  Step-parents
  In-laws
Failure in school
History of ineffective relationship with own
    parents (CLSE)
History of abusive relationships (CLSE)
Unrealistic expectations of child by parent
    (CLSE)
Unrealistic expectations of self (CLSE)
Unrealistic expectations of parent by child
    (CLSE)
Parental rejection (CLSE)
Overpassivity (CLSE)
Inconsistent punishment (CLSE)
Legal difficulties
Institutionalization
  Mental health facility
  Jail
  Orphanage
  Halfway house
Cultural Influences
  Ethnic group
  Minority
Drug/alcohol abuse by self or family member

Maturational

Infant/toddler/preschool
  Lack of stimulation (CLSE)

Separation from parents/significant others
(CLSE)
Restriction of activity (CLSE)
Inadequate parental support (CLSE)
Inability to trust significant other (CLSE)
School age
Loss of significant others
Failure to achieve grade level objectives
Loss of peer group
Adolescent
Loss of independence and autonomy
Disruption of peer relationships
Disruption in body image
Interruption of intellectual achievement
Loss of significant others
Career choices
Middle age
Signs of graying
Menopause
Career pressures
Elderly
Losses (people, function, financial, retirement)

Chronic Low Self-esteem

DEFINITION

Chronic Low Self-esteem: The state in which an individual experiences a long-standing negative self-evaluation about self or capabilities.

DEFINING CHARACTERISTICS*

Major (80%–100%)

Long-standing or chronic:
Self-negating verbalization

* Norris J, Kunes-Connell M: Self esteem disturbance: A
clinical validation study. In McLane A (ed): Classification
of Nursing Diagnoses: Proceedings of the Seventh Conference. St Louis, CV Mosby, 1987

Expressions of shame/guilt
Evaluates self as unable to deal with events
Rationalizes away/rejects positive feedback
and exaggerates negative feedback about
self
Hesitant to try new things/situations

Minor (50%–79%)

Frequent lack of success in work or other life
events
Overly conforming, dependent on opinions of
others
Lack of eye contact
Nonassertive/passive
Indecisive
Excessively seeks reassurance

ETIOLOGICAL, CONTRIBUTING, RISK FACTORS

See Self-esteem Disturbance.

Situational Low Self-esteem

DEFINITION

Situational Low Self-esteem: The state in which an individual who previously had positive self-esteem experiences negative feelings about self in response to an event (loss, change).

Author's Note:
Although situational low self-esteem is an episodic event, repeated occurrences and/or the continuation of these negative self-appraisals over time can lead to chronic low self-esteem (Willard).

DEFINING CHARACTERISTICS*

Major (80%–100%)

Episodic occurrence of negative self-appraisal in response to life events in a person with a previous positive self-evaluation

Verbalization of negative feelings about self (helplessness, uselessness)

Minor (50%–79%)

Self-negating verbalizations

Expressions of shame/guilt

Evaluates self as unable to handle situations/ events

Difficulty making decisions

ETIOLOGICAL, CONTRIBUTING, RISK FACTORS

See Self-esteem disturbance.

Self-harm, Potential for†

DEFINITION

Potential for Self-harm: The state in which an individual is at risk for inflicting direct harm on himself/ herself.

---

* Norris J, Kunes-Connell M: Self esteem disturbance: A clinical validation study. In McLane A (ed): Classification of Nursing Diagnoses: Proceedings of the Seventh Conference. St Louis, CV Mosby, 1987

† This diagnostic category is not currently on the NANDA list but has been included for clarity or usefulness.

DEFINING CHARACTERISTICS

Major (Must Be Present)

Suicidal ideation

Minor (May Be Present)

Severe stress
Depression
Hallucinations/delusions
Hostility
Substance abuse
Low self-esteem
Hopelessness
Acute agitation
Poor impulse control
Lack of a support system
Helplessness

ETIOLOGICAL, CONTRIBUTING, RISK FACTORS

Potential for self-harm can occur as a response to a variety of health problems, situations, and conflicts. Some sources are the following:

Pathophysiological

Terminal illness
Chronic illness (*e.g.,* diabetes, hypertension)
Alcoholism
Organic mental disorder
Ingestion of prescribed or nonprescribed drugs

Treatment-related

Dialysis
Insulin injections or any ongoing treatments
Cancer chemotherapy/radiation

Situational (Personal, Environmental)

Parental/marital conflict
Job loss
Divorce/separation
Threatened or actual financial loss
Alcoholism/drug abuse in family
Wish to reunite with loved one who has died
Depression
Death of significant other
Loss of status, prestige
Inadequate coping skills
Someone leaving home
Child abuse
Threat of abandonment by significant other

Maturational

Adolescent
    Separation from family
    Peer pressure
    Role changes
    Identity crisis
    Loss of significant support person
Adult
    Marital conflict
    Parenting
    Loss of family member
    Role changes
Elderly
    Retirement
    Social isolation
    Loss of spouse

Sensory–Perceptual Alteration

DEFINITION

Sensory–Perceptual Alteration: The state in which an individual/group experiences or is at risk of experiencing a change in the amount, pattern, or interpretation of incoming stimuli.

The category Sensory–Perceptual Alteration has six subcategories: visual, auditory, kinesthetic, gustatory, tactile, and olfactory.

When an individual has a visual or hearing deficit, how does the nurse intervene with the diagnosis Sensory–Perceptual Alteration: visual related to effects of glaucoma? What would the outcome criteria be? The nurse should assess for the individual's response to the visual loss and specifically label the response, not the deficit. Examples of responses to sensory deficits may be the following:

Visual
   Potential for injury
   Self-care deficit
Auditory
   Impaired communicaton
   Social isolation
Kinesthetic
   Potential for injury
Olfactory
   Altered nutrition
Tactile
   Potential for injury
Gustatory
   Altered nutrition

Altered Thought Processes describes an individual with altered cognition and perception influenced by coping problems. It differs from Sensory–Perceptual Alteration, which describes an individual with altered perception and cognition influenced by physiological functions and stimuli from the environment.

DEFINING CHARACTERISTICS

Major (Must Be Present)

Inaccurate interpretation of environmental
      stimuli
or
Negative change in amount or pattern of
      incoming stimuli

Minor (May Be Present)

Disoriented about time or place
Disoriented about people

Altered problem-solving ability
Altered behavior or communication pattern
Sleep pattern disturbances
Restlessness
Reports auditory or visual hallucinations
Fear
Anxiety
Apathy

ETIOLOGICAL, CONTRIBUTING, RISK FACTORS

Many factors in an individual's life can contribute to sensory–perceptual alterations. Some common factors are listed below.

Pathophysiological

Sensory organ alterations (visual, gustatory, auditory, olfactory, and tactile deficits)
Neurological alterations
  Cerebrovascular   Neuropathies
    accident (CVA)
  Encephalitis/
    meningitis
Metabolic alterations
  Fluid and electrolyte   Acidosis
    imbalance   Alkalosis
  Elevated blood urea
    nitrogen (BUN)
Impaired oxygen transport
  Cerebral   Respiratory
  Cardiac   Anemia
Musculoskeletal changes
  Paraplegia   Quadriplegia

Treatment-related

Amputation
Medications (sedatives, tranquilizers)
Surgery (glaucoma, cataract, detached retina)
Physical isolation (reverse isolation, communicable disease, prison)
Radiation therapy
Immobility
Mobility restrictions (bed rest, traction, casts, Stryker frame, Circoelectric bed)

Situational (Personal, Environmental)

> Social isolation (patient with terminal or
>   infectious disease)
> Pain
> Stress
> Environment ("noise pollution")

Sexuality Patterns, Altered

Sexual Dysfunction

DEFINITION

Altered Sexuality Patterns: The state in which an individual experiences or is at risk of experiencing a change in sexual health.

> **Author's Note:**
> Altered Sexuality Patterns is a broad diagnostic category that encompasses sexual identity, sexuality, and sexual function. Sexual Dysfunction describes dissatisfaction with sexual function.
>
> According to the World Health Organization, sexual health is "the integration of somatic, emotional, intellectual, and social aspects of sexual being in ways that are enriching and that enhance personality, communication, and love."

DEFINING CHARACTERISTICS

Major (Must Be Present)

> Identification of sexual difficulties, limitations, or
>   changes

ETIOLOGICAL, CONTRIBUTING, RISK FACTORS

Altered sexuality patterns can occur as a response to a variety of health problems, situations, and conflicts. Some common sources are indicated below.

Pathophysiological

Endocrine
    Diabetes mellitus
    Decreased hormone
        production
    Myxedema

    Hyperthyroidism
    Addison's disease
    Acromegaly

Genitourinary
    Chronic renal
        failure
    Premature or
        retarded
        ejaculation
    Priapism
    Chronic vaginal
        infection

    Decreased vaginal
        lubrication
    Vaginismus
    Altered structures
    Venereal disease

Neuromuscular and skeletal
    Arthritis
    Multiple sclerosis
    Amyotrophic lateral
        sclerosis

    Disturbances of the
        nerve supply to
        the brain,
        spinal cord,
        sensory nerves,
        and autonomic
        nerves

Cardiorespiratory
    Myocardial
        infarction
    Congestive heart
        failure
Cancer
Liver disease

    Peripheral vascular
        disorders
    Chronic respiratory
        disorders

Treatment-related

Medications
Radiation treatment
Altered self-concept from change in appearance
    (trauma, radical surgery)

Situational (Personal, Environmental)

Partner
  Unwilling
  Uninformed
  Abusive
  Not available
  Separated
  Divorced
Environment
  Unfamiliar
  No privacy
  Hospital
Stressors
  Job problems
  Financial worries
  Conflicting values
  Religious conflict
Lack of knowledge
Fatigue
Obesity
Pain
Alcohol ingestion
Drug abuse
Fear of sexual failure
Fear of pregnancy
Depression
Anxiety
Guilt
Fear of sexually transmitted disease

Maturational

Ineffective role models
Negative sexual teaching
Absence of sexual teaching
Aging (separation, isolation)

Sexual Dysfunction

DEFINITION

Sexual Dysfunction: The state in which an individual experiences or is at risk of experiencing a change in sexual function that is viewed as unrewarding or inadequate.

DEFINING CHARACTERISTICS

Major (Must Be Present)

Verbalization of problem with sexual function
or
Reports limitations on sexual performance
imposed by disease or therapy

Minor (May Be Present)

Fears future limitations on sexual performance
Misinformed about sexuality
Lacks knowledge about sexuality and sexual
function
Value conflicts involving sexual expression
(cultural, religious)
Altered relationship with significant other
Dissatisfaction with sex role (perceived or actual)

ETIOLOGICAL, CONTRIBUTING, RISK FACTORS

See Altered Sexuality Patterns.

Sleep Pattern Disturbance

DEFINITION

Sleep Pattern Disturbance: The state in which an individual experiences or is at risk of experiencing a change in the quantity or quality of his rest pattern as related to his biological and emotional needs.

DEFINING CHARACTERISTICS

Adults

Major (Must Be Present)

Difficulty falling or remaining asleep

Minor (May Be Present)

Fatigue on awakening or during the day
Dozing during the day
Agitation
Mood alterations

Children

Sleep disturbances in children are frequently related
to fear, enuresis, or inconsistent responses of parents
to the child's requests for changes in sleep rules, such
as requests to stay up late.

Reluctance to retire
Frequent awakening during the night
Desire to sleep with parents

ETIOLOGICAL, CONTRIBUTING, RISK FACTORS

Many factors in life can contribute to sleep pattern
disturbances. Some common factors are listed below.

Pathophysiological

Impaired oxygen transport
  Angina   Respiratory
  Peripheral   disorders
    arteriosclerosis   Circulatory
                                  disorders
Impaired elimination (bowel or bladder)
  Diarrhea   Retention
  Constipation   Dysuria
  Incontinence   Frequency
Impaired metabolism
  Hyperthyroidism   Hepatic disorders
  Gastric ulcers

Treatment-related

Immobility (imposed by casts, traction)
Medications
  Tranquilizers   Soporifics
  Sedatives   Monoamine oxidase
  Hypnotics   (MAO)
  Antidepressants   inhibitors

Antihypertensives	Anesthetics
Amphetamines	Barbiturates
Corticosteroids	

Situational (Personal, Environmental)

Lack of exercise
Pain
Anxiety response
Pregnancy
Life-style disruptions

Occupational	Sexual
Emotional	Financial
Social	

Environmental changes

Hospitalization	Travel
(noise,	
disturbing	
roommate,	
fear)	

Social Interactions, Impaired

DEFINITION

Impaired Social Interactions: The state in which an individual experiences or is at risk of experiencing negative, insufficient, or unsatisfactory responses from interactions.

DEFINING CHARACTERISTICS

Major (Must Be Present)

Reports inability to establish and/or maintain stable supportive relationships

Minor (May Be Present)

Lack of motivation
Severe anxiety

Dependent behavior
Hopelessness
Delusions/hallucinations
Disorganized thinking
Lack of self-care skills
Distractibility/inability to concentrate
Social isolation
Superficial relationships
Poor impulse control
Difficulty holding a job
Lack of self-esteem

ETIOLOGICAL, CONTRIBUTING, RISK FACTORS

Impaired social interactions can result from a variety of situations and health problems that are related to the inability to establish and maintain rewarding relationships. Some common sources are as follows:

Pathophysiological

Loss of body function
Hearing deficits
Mental retardation
Terminal illness
Loss of body part
Visual deficits
Speech impediments
Chronic illness (Crohn's disease, renal failure, epilepsy)

Treatment-related

Surgical disfigurement
Dialysis
Medication reaction

Situational (Personal, Environmental)

Depression
Language/cultural barriers
Social isolation
Lack of vocational skills
Substance abuse
Anxiety (phobias)

Divorce/death of spouse
Institutionalization
Thought disturbances

Maturational

Child/adolescent
    Altered appearance
    Speech impediments
    Separation from family
Adult
    Loss of ability to practice vocation
Elderly
    Death of spouse
    Retirement

Social Isolation

DEFINITION

Social Isolation: The state in which an individual or group experiences a need or desire for contact with others but is unable to make that contact.

Author's Note:

Social isolation is a negative state of aloneness. It is a subjective state that exists whenever a person says it does and is perceived as imposed by others. Social isolation is *not* the voluntary solitude that is necessary for personal renewal, nor is it the creative aloneness of the artist or the loneliness—and possible suffering—one may experience as a result of seeking individualism and independence (*e.g.,* moving to a new city, going away to college).

DEFINING CHARACTERISTICS

Since social isolation is a subjective state, all inferences made regarding a person's feelings of aloneness must be validated. Because the causes vary and people show their aloneness in different ways, there are no absolute cues to this diagnosis.

Major (Must Be Present)

Expressed feelings of aloneness and/or desire for more social contact

Minor (May Be Present)

Time passing slowly ("Mondays are so long for me.")
Inability to concentrate and make decisions
Feelings of uselessness
Doubts about ability to survive
Feelings of rejection
Behavior changes
  Increased irritability or restlessness
  Underactivity (physical or verbal)
  Inability to make decisions
  Increased signs and symptoms of illness (a change from previous state of good health)
  Appearing depressed, anxious, or angry
  Postponing important decision-making
  Failure to interact with others nearby
  Sleep disturbance (too much or insomnia)
  Change in eating habits (overeating or anorexia)

ETIOLOGICAL, CONTRIBUTING, RISK FACTORS

A state of social isolation can result from a variety of situations and health problems that are related to a loss of established relationships or to a failure to generate these relationships. Some common sources follow.

Pathophysiological

Obesity
Cancer (disfiguring surgery of head or neck, superstitions of others)
Physical handicaps (paraplegia, amputation, arthritis, hemiplegia)

Emotional handicaps (extreme anxiety,
depression, paranoia, phobias)
Incontinence (embarrassment, odor)
Communicable diseases (acquired
immunodeficiency syndrome [AIDS],
hepatitis)

Situational (Personal, Environmental)

Death of a significant other
Divorce
Extreme poverty
Hospitalization or terminal illness (dying
process)
Moving to another culture (*e.g.,* unfamiliar
language)
Drug or alcohol addiction
Homosexuality
Loss of usual means of transportation

Maturational

Child
In protective isolation or with a
communicable disease
Elderly
Sensory losses
Motor losses
Loss of significant others

Spiritual Distress

DEFINITION

Spiritual Distress: The state in which an individual
or group experiences or is at risk of experiencing a
disturbance in the belief or value system that provides
strength, hope, and meaning to one's life.

DEFINING CHARACTERISTICS

Major (Must Be Present)

Experiences a disturbance in belief system

Minor (May Be Present)

Questions credibility of belief system
Demonstrates discouragement or despair
Is unable to practice usual religious rituals
Has ambivalent feelings (doubts) about beliefs
Expresses that he has no reason for living
Feels a sense of spiritual emptiness
Shows emotional detachment from self and
    others
Expresses concern—anger, resentment, fear—
    over the meaning of life, suffering, death
Requests spiritual assistance for a disturbance in
    belief system

ETIOLOGICAL, CONTRIBUTING, RISK FACTORS

Pathophysiological

Loss of body part or function
Terminal illness
Debilitating disease
Pain
Trauma
Miscarriage, stillbirth

Treatment-related

Abortion	Isolation
Surgery	Amputation
Blood transfusion	Medications
Dietary restrictions	Medical procedures

Situational (Personal, Environmental)

Death or illness of significant other
Embarrassment at practicing spiritual rituals
Hospital barriers to practicing spiritual rituals

Intensive-care	Lack of privacy
restrictions	Lack of availability
Confinement to bed	of special
or room	foods/diet

Beliefs opposed by family, peers, health care
    providers
Childbirth
Divorce, separation from loved ones

Thought Processes, Altered

DEFINITION

Altered Thought Processes: The state in which an individual experiences a disruption in such mental activities as conscious thought, reality orientation, problem-solving, judgment, and comprehension related to coping.

Author's Note:

Altered Thought Processes is the state in which an individual experiences a disruption in such mental activities as conscious thought, reality orientation, problem-solving, judgment, and comprehension related to coping (personality, mental) disorders. Cognitive function is influenced by physiological functions, stimuli from the environment, and the person's emotional status. Altered Thought Processes describes an individual with altered cognition and perception influenced by coping problems. It differs from Sensory–Perceptual Alterations, which describes an individual with altered perception and cognition influenced by physiological functions and stimuli from the environment.

DEFINING CHARACTERISTICS

Major (Must Be Present)

Inaccurate interpretation of stimuli, internal and/or external

Minor (May Be Present)

Cognitive deficits, including abstraction, memory deficits
Suspiciousness
Delusions

Hallucinations
Distractibility
Lack of consensual validation
Language
Confusion/disorientation

ETIOLOGICAL, CONTRIBUTING, RISK FACTORS
Pathophysiological

Personality and mental disorders related to
Alteration in biochemical compounds
Genetic disorder
Progressive dementia

Situational (Personal, Environmental)

Depression or anxiety
Substance abuse (alcohol, drugs)
Fear of the unknown
Actual loss (of control, routine, income,
significant others, familiar object or
surroundings)
Emotional trauma
Rejection or negative appraisal by others
Negative response from others
Isolation
Unclear communication

Maturational*

Adolescent
Peer pressure
Conflict
Separation
Adult
Marital conflict
Family additions or deaths
Elderly
Isolation

* These situational and maturational factors should not
be considered causative or contributive unless they are present in an individual with a history of coping disorders.

Tissue Integrity, Impaired

Skin Integrity, Impaired

Oral Mucous Membrane, Altered

DEFINITION

Impaired Tissue Integrity: The state in which an individual experiences or is at risk for damage to the integumentary, corneal, or mucous membranous tissues.

Author's Note:

Impaired Tissue Integrity is the broad category under which the more specific diagnostic categories of Impaired Skin Integrity and Altered Oral Mucous Membranes fall. Since tissue is composed of epithelium and connective, muscle, and nervous tissue, Impaired Tissue Integrity correctly describes some pressure ulcers that are deeper than dermal. Impaired Skin Integrity should be used to describe potential or actual disruptions of epidermal and dermal tissue only. If an individual is at risk for damage to corneal tissue, the nurse can use the diagnosis Potential Impaired Corneal Tissue Integrity related to; for example: to corneal drying and reduced lacrimal production secondary to unconscious state. If an individual is immobile and multiple systems—respiratory, circulatory, musculoskeletal, and integumentary—are threatened, the nurse can use Potential for Disuse Syndrome to describe the entire situation.

DEFINING CHARACTERISTICS

Major (Must Be Present)

Disruptions of corneal, integumentary, or mucous membranous tissue or invasion of body structure (incision, dermal ulcer, corneal ulcer, oral lesion)

Minor (May Be Present)

Lesions (primary, secondary)
Edema
Erythema
Dry mucous membrane
Leukoplakia
Coated tongue

ETIOLOGICAL, CONTRIBUTING, RISK FACTORS

Pathophysiological

Autoimmune alterations
   Lupus   Scleroderma
      erythematosus
Metabolic and endocrine alterations
   Diabetes mellitus   Jaundice
   Hepatitis   Cancer
   Cirrhosis   Thyroid dysfunction
   Renal failure
Nutritional alterations
   Obesity   Emaciation
   Dehydration   Malnutrition
   Edema
Impaired oxygen transport
   Peripheral vascular   Anemia
      alterations   Cardiopulmonary
   Venous stasis   disorders
   Arteriosclerosis
Medications (corticosteroid therapy)
Psoriasis
Eczema
Infections
   Bacterial (impetigo, folliculitis, cellulitis)

Viral (herpes zoster [shingles], herpes simplex,
gingivitis, acquired immunodeficiency
syndrome [AIDS])
Fungal (ringworm [dermatophytosis], athlete's
foot, vaginitis)
Dental caries/periodontal disease

Treatment-related

NPO status
Therapeutic extremes in body temperature
Therapeutic irradiation
Surgery
Drug therapy (local and systemic)
  Corticosteroids
Imposed immobility related to sedation
Mechanical trauma
  Therapeutic fixation devices
    Wired jaw
    Traction
    Casts
    Orthopedic devices/braces
  Inflatable or foam "donuts"
  Tourniquets
  Footboards
  Restraints
  Dressings, tape, solutions
  External urinary catheters
  Nasogastric tubes
  Endotracheal tubes
  Oral prostheses/braces
  Contact lenses

Situational (Personal, Environmental)

Chemical trauma
  Excretions   Noxious agents/
  Secretions   substances
Environmental
  Radiation—sunburn   Bites (insect,
  Temperature   animal)
  Humidity   Inhalants
  Parasites   Poison plants
Immobility
  Related to pain; fatigue; motivation; cognitive,
    sensory, or motor deficits

Personal
  Allergies
  Inadequate personal habits (hygiene/dental/
      dietary/sleep)
  Body build/weight distribution/bony
      prominences/muscle mass/range of
      motion/joint mobility
  Stress
  Occupation
  Pregnancy

Maturational

Infants/children
  Diaper rash
  Childhood diseases (chickenpox)
Elderly
  Dry skin
  Thin skin
  Loss of skin elasticity
  Loss of subcutaneous tissue

Skin Integrity, Impaired

DEFINITION

Impaired Skin Integrity: The state in which an individual experiences or is at risk for damage to the epidermal and dermal tissue.

DEFINING CHARACTERISTICS

Major (Must Be Present)

  Disruptions of epidermal and dermal tissue

Minor (May Be Present)

  Denuded skin
  Erythema
  Lesions (primary, secondary)
  Pruritus

ETIOLOGICAL, CONTRIBUTING, RISK FACTORS

See *Impaired Tissue Integrity.*

Oral Mucous Membrane, Altered

DEFINITION

Altered Oral Mucous Membrane: The state in which an individual experiences or is at risk of experiencing disruptions in the oral cavity.

DEFINING CHARACTERISTICS

Major (Must Be Present)

Disrupted oral mucous membranes

Minor (May Be Present)

Coated tongue
Xerostomia (dry
    mouth)
Stomatitis
Oral tumors
Oral lesions

Leukoplakia
Edema
Hemorrhagic
    gingivitis
Purulent drainage

ETIOLOGICAL, CONTRIBUTING, RISK FACTORS

Pathophysiological

Diabetes mellitus
Oral cancer
Periodontal disease
Infection
    Herpes simplex   Gingivitis

Treatment-related

NPO 24 hours
Radiation to head or neck
Prolonged use of corticosteroids or other
        immunosuppressives
Use of antineoplastic drugs
Endotrachial intubation
Nasogastric intubation

Situational (Personal, Environmental)

Chemical trauma
  Acidic foods   Alcohol
  Drugs   Tobacco
  Noxious agents
Mechanical trauma
  Broken or jagged   Ill-fitting dentures
    teeth   Braces
Malnutrition
Dehydration
Mouth breathing
Inadequate oral hygiene
Lack of knowledge
Fractured mandible

Tissue Perfusion, Altered: (Specify)

DEFINITION

Altered Tissue Perfusion: The state in which an individual experiences or is at risk of experiencing a decrease in nutrition and respiration at the cellular level because of a decrease in capillary blood supply.

Altered Peripheral Tissue Perfusion: The state in which an individual experiences or is at risk of experiencing a decrease in nutrition and respiration at the peripheral cellular level because of a decrease in capillary blood supply.

Author's Note:
This diagnostic category is restricted in use to represent only diminished peripheral tissue perfusion situations in which nurses prescribe definitive treatment to reduce, eliminate, or prevent the problem. In the other situations of diminished cardiopulmo-
(Continued)

Author's Note (Continued)
nary, cerebral, renal, or gastrointestinal tissue perfusion, the nurse should focus on the functional abilities of the individual that are or may be compromised because of the decreased tissue perfusion. The nurse should also monitor to detect for physiological complications of decreased tissue perfusion and label these situations as collaborative problems. The following illustrates examples of a compromised functional health problem (nursing diagnosis) and a potential complication (collaborative problem) for an individual with compromised cerebral tissue perfusion:

Potential for Injury related to vertigo secondary to recent head injury (nursing diagnosis)

Potential Complication: Increased Intracranial Pressure (collaborative problem)

Refer to Chapter 2 of Carpenito LJ: Nursing Diagnosis: Application to Clinical Practice, 3rd ed. Philadelphia, JB Lippincott, 1989 for additional information on collaborative problems. For additional examples of nursing diagnoses and collaborative problems grouped under medical conditions, refer to Section II of this handbook.

DEFINING CHARACTERISTICS*

Major (Must Be Present)

Presence of one of the following types:
Claudication   Aching pain
Rest pain
Diminished or absent arterial pulses

* Tissue perfusion is dependent upon many physical and physiological factors within the systems of the body and in the structures and functions of the cells. When an alteration in peripheral tissue perfusion exists, the nurse must take into account the nature of the alteration in perfusion. The two major components of the peripheral vascular system are the arterial and the venous systems. Signs, symptoms, etiologies, and nursing interventions are different for problems occurring in each of these two systems and are therefore addressed separately when appropriate.

Skin color changes
  Pallor (arterial)   Reactive hyperemia
  Cyanosis (venous)   (arterial)
Skin temperature changes
  Cooler (arterial)   Warmer (venous)
Decreased blood pressure changes (arterial)
Capillary refill less than three seconds (arterial)

Minor (May Be Present)

Edema (venous)
Loss of sensory function (arterial)
Loss of motor function (arterial)
Trophic tissue changes (arterial)
  Hard, thick nails
  Loss of hair
  Lack of lanugo (newborn)

ETIOLOGICAL, CONTRIBUTING, RISK FACTORS

Pathophysiological

Vascular disorders
  Arteriosclerosis   Leriche syndrome
  Hypertension   Raynaud's disease/
  Aneurysm   syndrome
  Arterial thrombosis   Varicosities
  Deep vein   Buerger's disease
    thrombosis   Sickle cell crisis
  Collagen vascular   Cirrhosis
    disease   Alcoholism
  Rheumatoid
    arthritis
Diabetes Mellitus
Hypotension
  Sympathetic stress response (vasospasm/
    vasoconstriction)
Blood dyscrasias (platelet disorders)
Renal failure
Cancer/tumor

Treatment-related

Immobilization
Presence of invasive lines

Pressure sites/constriction (Ace bandages, stockings)
Medications (diuretics, tranquilizers, anticoagulants)
Anesthesia
Blood vessel trauma or compression

Situational (Personal, Environmental)

Pregnancy
Heredity
Obesity
Diet (hyperlipidemia)
Anorexia/Malnutrition
Dehydration
Dependent venous pooling
Hypothermia
Frequent exposure to vibrating tools/equipment
Tobacco use
Exercise

Maturational

Neonate
    Immature peripheral circulation
    Rh incompatibility (erythroblastosis fetalis)
    Hypothermia
Elderly
    Sensory–perceptual changes
    Atherosclerotic plaques
    Capillary fragility

Unilateral Neglect

DEFINITION

Unilateral Neglect: The state in which an individual is unable to attend to or "ignores" the hemiplegic side of his body and/or objects, persons, or sounds on the affected side of his environment.

DEFINING CHARACTERISTICS

Major (Must Be Present)

Neglect of involved body parts and/or extrapersonal space and/or denial of the existence of the affected limb or side of the body

Minor (May Be Present)

Left homonymous hemianopsia
Difficulty with spatial–perceptual tasks
Hemiplegia (usually left side)

ETIOLOGICAL, CONTRIBUTING, RISK FACTORS

Pathophysiological

Neurological disease/damage
Cerebrovascular accident (CVA)
Cerebral tumors
Brain injury/trauma
Cerebral aneurysms

Urinary Elimination, Altered Patterns of

Maturational Enuresis*

Functional Incontinence

Reflex Incontinence

* This diagnostic category is not currently on the NANDA list but has been included for clarity or usefulness.

Stress Incontinence

Total Incontinence

Urge Incontinence

Urinary Retention

Author's Note:

All of these categories pertain to urine elimination, not urine formulation. Anuria, oliguria, and renal failure should be labeled collaborative problems, such as Potential Complication: Anuria. Altered Patterns of Urinary Elimination represents a broad diagnosis, probably too broad for clinical use. It is recommended that a more specific diagnostic category such as Stress Incontinence be used instead. When the etiological or contributing factors have not been identified for incontinence, the diagnosis can temporarily be written Incontinence related to unknown etiology.

DEFINITION

Altered Patterns of Urinary Elimination: The state in which an individual experiences or is at risk of experiencing urinary elimination dysfunction.

DEFINING CHARACTERISTICS

Major (Must Be Present)

Reports or experiences a urinary elimination
    problem, such as

Urgency	Dribbling
Frequency	Bladder distention
Hesitancy	Incontinence
Nocturia	Large residual urine
Enuresis	volumes

ETIOLOGICAL, CONTRIBUTING, RISK FACTORS

Pathophysiological

Congenital urinary tract anomolies
Strictures
Hypospadias
Epispadias
Ureterocele
Bladder neck contractures
Megalocystis (large-capacity bladder without tone)

Disorders of the urinary tract
Infection
Trauma
Urethritis
Calculi
Carcinoma

Neurogenic disorders or injuries
Cord injury/tumor/infection
Brain injury/tumor/infection
Cerebrovascular accident
Demyelinating diseases
Multiple sclerosis
Diabetic neuropathy
Alcoholic neuropathy
Tabes dorsalis
Parkinsonism

Prostatic enlargement
Estrogen deficiency
Atrophic vaginitis
Herpes zoster
Atrophic urethritis

Treatment-related

Surgical
Postprostatectomy
Extensive pelvic dissection

Diagnostic instrumentation
General or spinal anesthesia
Drug therapy (iatrogenic)
Antihistamines
Epinephrine
Anticholinergics
Sedatives
Immunosuppressant therapy
Diuretics
Tranquilizers
Muscle relaxants

Post–indwelling catheters

Situational (Personal, Environmental)

Loss of perineal tissue
Obesity
Childbirth

Aging
Recent substantial
weight loss
Irritation to perineal area
Sexual activity   Poor personal
                                    hygiene

Pregnancy
Inability to communicate needs
Fecal impaction
Dehydration
Stress or fear
Decreased attention to bladder cues
Depression   Confusion
Intentional suppression (self-induced
deconditioning)
Environmental barriers to bathroom
Distant toilets   Bed too high
Poor lighting   Siderails
Unfamiliar
surroundings
Impaired mobility

Maturational

Child
Small bladder capacity
Lack of motivation
Elderly
Motor and sensory losses
Loss of muscle tone
Inability to communicate needs
Depression

Maturational Enuresis*

DEFINITION

Maturational Enuresis: The state in which a child experiences involuntary voiding during sleep, which is not pathophysiological in origin.

* This diagnostic category is not currently on the NANDA list but has been included for clarity or usefulness.

DEFINING CHARACTERISTICS

Major (Must Be Present)

Reports or demonstrates episodes of involuntary voiding during sleep

ETIOLOGICAL, CONTRIBUTING, RISK FACTORS

Situational (Personal, Environmental)

Stressors (school, siblings)
Inattention to bladder cues
Unfamiliar surroundings

Maturational

Child
Small bladder capacity
Lack of motivation
Attention-seeking behavior

Functional Incontinence

DEFINITION

Functional Incontinence: The state in which an individual experiences difficulty in reaching or inability to reach the toilet prior to urination because of environmental barriers, disorientation, and physical limitations.

DEFINING CHARACTERISTICS

Major (Must Be Present)

Incontinence before or during an attempt to reach the toilet

ETIOLOGICAL, CONTRIBUTING, RISK FACTORS

Pathophysiological

Neurogenic disorders
  Brain injury/tumor/infection
  Cerebrovascular accident
  Demyelinating diseases
  Multiple sclerosis
  Alcoholic neuropathy
  Parkinsonism
Progressive dementia

Treatment-related

Drug therapy (iatrogenic)
  Antihistamines
  Epinephrine
  Anticholinergics
  Sedatives
  Immunosuppressant therapy
  Diuretics
  Tranquilizers
  Muscle relaxants

Situational (Personal, Environmental)

Impaired Mobility
Stress or fear
Decreased attention to bladder cues
  Depression
  Confusion
  Intentional suppression (self-induced
      deconditioning)
Environmental barriers to bathroom
  Distant toilets
  Poor lighting
  Unfamiliar surroundings
  Bed too high
  Siderails

Maturational

Elderly
  Motor and sensory losses
  Loss of muscle tone
  Inability to communicate needs
  Depression

Reflex Incontinence

DEFINITION

Reflex Incontinence: The state in which an individual experiences an involuntary loss of urine caused by damage to the spinal cord between the cortical and sacral (S1–S3) bladder centers.

DEFINING CHARACTERISTICS

Major (Must Be Present)

Uninhibited bladder contractions
Involuntary reflexes produce spontaneous
    voiding
Partial or complete loss of sensation of bladder
    fullness or urge to void

ETIOLOGICAL, CONTRIBUTING, RISK FACTORS

Pathophysiological

Cord injury/tumor/infection

Stress Incontinence

DEFINITION

Stress Incontinence: The state in which an individual experiences an immediate involuntary loss of urine upon an increase in intra-abdominal pressure.

DEFINING CHARACTERISTICS

Major (Must Be Present)

The individual reports
    Loss of urine (usually less than 50 ml)
        occurring with increased abdominal
        pressure from standing, sneezing, or
        coughing

ETIOLOGICAL, CONTRIBUTING, RISK FACTORS

Pathophysiological

Congenital urinary tract anomalies
    Strictures
    Hypospadias
    Epispadias
    Ureterocele
    Bladder neck contractures
    Megalocystis (large-capacity bladder without tone)
Disorders of the urinary tract
    Infection
    Trauma
    Urethritis
Estrogen deficiency
    Atrophic vaginitis
    Atrophic urethritis

Situational (Personal, Environmental)

Loss of perineal tissue
    Obesity
    Aging
    Recent substantial weight loss
    Childbirth
Irritation to perineal area
    Sexual activity
    Poor personal hygiene
Pregnancy
Stress or fear

Maturational

Elderly
    Loss of muscle tone

Total Incontinence

DEFINITION

Total Incontinence: The state in which an individual experiences continuous, unpredictable loss of urine.

> **Author's Note:**
> This category is used only after the other types of incontinence have been ruled out.

DEFINING CHARACTERISTICS

Major (Must Be Present)

Constant flow of urine without distention
Nocturia more than two times during sleep
Incontinence refractory to other treatments

Minor (May Be Present)

Unaware of bladder cues to void
Unaware of incontinence

ETIOLOGICAL, CONTRIBUTING, RISK FACTORS

Pathophysiological

Congenital urinary tract anomalies
    Strictures
    Hypospadias
    Epispadias
    Ureterocele
    Megalocystis (large-capacity bladder without tone)
Disorders of the urinary tract
    Infection
    Trauma
    Urethritis
Neurogenic disorders or injury
    Cord injury/tumor/infection
    Brain injury/tumor/infection
    Cerebrovascular accident
    Demyelinating diseases
    Multiple sclerosis
    Diabetic neuropathy
    Alcoholic neuropathy
    Tabes dorsalis

Treatment-related

Surgical
  Postprostatectomy
  Extensive pelvic dissection
General or spinal anesthesia
Post–indwelling catheters

Situational (Personal, Environmental)

Inability to communicate needs
Dehydration
Stress or fear
Decreased attention to bladder cues
  Depression
  Confusion

Maturational

Elderly
  Motor and sensory losses
  Loss of muscle tone
  Inability to communicate needs
  Depression

Urge Incontinence

DEFINITION

Urge Incontinence: The state in which an individual experiences an involuntary loss of urine associated with a strong sudden desire to void.

DEFINING CHARACTERISTICS

Major (Must Be Present)

Urgency followed by incontinence

ETIOLOGICAL, CONTRIBUTING, RISK FACTORS

Pathophysiological

Disorders of the urinary tract
  Infection

Trauma
Urethritis
Neurogenic disorders or injury
    Brain injury/tumor/infection
    Cerebrovascular accident
    Demyelinating diseases
    Diabetic neuropathy
    Alcoholic neuropathy
    Parkinsonism

Treatment-related

Diagnostic instrumentation
General or spinal anesthesia
Post–indwelling catheters

Situational (Personal, Environmental)

Loss of perineal tissue
    Obesity
    Aging
    Recent substantial weight loss
    Childbirth
Irritation to perineal area
    Sexual activity
    Poor personal hygiene
Intentional suppression (self-induced
    deconditioning)

Maturational

Child
    Small bladder capacity

Urinary Retention

DEFINITION

Urinary Retention: The state in which an individual experiences a chronic inability to void followed by involuntary voiding (overflow incontinence).

DEFINING CHARACTERISTICS

Major (Must Be Present)

Bladder distention (not related to acute, reversible etiology)
or
Bladder distention with small frequent voids or dribbling (overflow incontinence)
100 ml or more residual urine

Minor (May Be Present)

The individual states that it feels as though the bladder is not empty after voiding.

ETIOLOGICAL, CONTRIBUTING, RISK FACTORS

Pathophysiological

Congenital urinary tract anomalies
  Strictures
  Ureterocele
  Bladder neck contractures
  Megalocystis (large-capacity bladder without tone)
Neurogenic disorders or injury
  Cord injury/tumor/infection
  Brain injury/tumor/infection
  Cerebrovascular accident
  Demyelinating diseases
  Multiple sclerosis
  Diabetic neuropathy

Alcoholic neuropathy
Tabes dorsalis
Prostatic enlargement

Treatment-related

Surgical
Postprostatectomy
Extensive pelvic dissection
Diagnostic instrumentation
General or spinal anesthesia
Drug therapy (iatrogenic)
Antihistamines
Epinephrine
Anticholinergics
Theophylline
Isoproterenol
Post–indwelling catheters

Situational (Personal, Environmental)

Loss of perineal tissue
Obesity
Aging
Recent substantial weight loss
Childbirth
Irritation to perineal area
Sexual activity
Poor personal hygiene
Pregnancy
Inability to communicate needs
Fecal impaction
Dehydration
Stress or fear
Decreased attention to bladder cues
Depression
Confusion
Intentional suppression (self-induced
deconditioning)
Environmental barriers to bathroom
Distant toilets
Poor lighting
Unfamiliar surroundings
Bed too high
Siderails

Maturational

Child
  Small bladder capacity
  Lack of motivation
Elderly
  Motor and sensory losses
  Loss of muscle tone
  Inability to communicate needs
  Depression

Violence, Potential for

DEFINITION

Potential for Violence: The state in which an individual is or may be assaultive toward others or the environment.

Author's Note:
This diagnostic category can be made more specific by adding Potential for Violence directed at others or self-directed. Potential for Self-harm has been added by the author to describe individuals at risk for self-inflicted injuries; thus, the descriptor *self-directed* is not needed. Therefore, the content for Potential for Violence will focus exclusively on violence directed at others.

DEFINING CHARACTERISTICS

Major (Must Be Present)

Presence of risk factors (See also Etiological, Contributing, Risk Factors.)

ETIOLOGICAL, CONTRIBUTING, RISK FACTORS

Pathophysiological

Temporal lobe epilepsy
Progressive central nervous system deterioration
    (brain tumor)
Head injury
Hormonal imbalance
Viral encephalopathy
Mental retardation
Minimal brain dysfunction
Toxic response to alcohol or drugs
Mania

Treatment-related

Toxic reaction to medication

Situational (Personal, Environmental)

History of overt aggressive acts
Increase in stressors within a short period
Physical immobility
Suicidal behavior
Environmental controls
Perceived threat to self-esteem
Hallucination
Argumentive
Acute agitation
Suspiciousness
Persecutory delusions
Verbal threats of physical assault
Low frustration tolerance
Poor impulse control
Feelings of helplessness
Excessively controlled, inflexible
Fear of the unknown
Response to catastrophic event
Rage reaction
Misperceived messages from others
Antisocial character
Response to dysfunctional family throughout
    developmental stages

Dysfunctional communication patterns
Drug or alcohol abuse

Maturational

Adolescent
    Role identity
    Peer pressure
    Separation from family

Section II

Diagnostic Clusters
(Medical Diagnostic
Categories With
Associated Nursing
Diagnoses and
Collaborative Problems)

Medical Diagnoses

Cardiovascular/ Hematologic/Peripheral Vascular Disorders

Cardiac Conditions

ANGINA PECTORIS

Nursing Diagnoses*

Altered Comfort: Chest Pain related to effects of cardiac ischemia

Fear related to present status and unknown future

Sleep Pattern Disturbances related to treatments and environment

Potential Constipation related to bed rest, change in life-style, and medications

Activity Intolerance related to fear of recurrent angina

Potential Self-concept Disturbance related to perceived or actual role changes

Possible Impaired Home Maintenance Management related to angina or fear of angina

Potential Altered Family Processes related to impaired ability of person to assume role responsibilities

Potential Sexual Dysfunction related to fear of angina and altered self-concept

Grieving related to actual or perceived losses secondary to cardiac condition

Potential Altered Health Maintenance related to insufficient knowledge of: (specify)

* List includes nursing diagnoses that may be associated with the medical diagnosis.

Examples:
    Condition   Diet
    Home activities   Medications

CONGESTIVE HEART FAILURE WITH PULMONARY EDEMA

Collaborative Problems

Potential Complication*:   *Deep vein thrombosis*
Potential Complication*:   *Severe hypoxia*

Nursing Diagnoses

Activity Intolerance related to insufficient oxygen for activities of daily living

Altered Nutrition: Less Than Body Requirements related to nausea; anorexia secondary to venous congestion of gastrointestinal tract and fatigue

Altered Peripheral Tissue Perfusion related to venous congestion

Anxiety related to breathlessness

Fear related to progressive nature of condition

Potential Impaired Home Maintenance related to inability to perform activities of daily living secondary to breathlessness and fatigue

(Specify) Self-care Deficit related to dyspnea and fatigue

Sleep Pattern Disturbance related to nocturnal dyspnea and inability to assume usual sleep position

Potential Fluid Volume Excess: Edema related to compensatory kidney mechanisms

Potential Altered Health Maintenance related to insufficient knowledge of: (specify)

Examples:
Low-salt diet	Activity program
Drug therapy	Signs and
(diuretic,	symptoms of
digitalis)	complications

* Potential complications are collaborative problems, not nursing diagnoses.

ENDOCARDITIS, PERICARDITIS
(Rheumatic, Infectious)

See also Corticosteroid Therapy.
If child, see Rheumatic Fever.

Collaborative Problems

Potential Complications:

Congestive heart
  failure
Valve stenosis
Cerebrovascular
  accident (CVA)

Emboli (pulmonary,
  cerebral, renal,
  splenic, heart)
Cardiac tamponade

Nursing Diagnoses

Activity Intolerance related to insufficient
  oxygenation secondary to decreased cardiac
  output
Potential Altered Respiratory Function related to
  decreased respiratory depth secondary to
  pain
Acute Pain related to friction rub and
  inflammation process
Potential Altered Health Maintenance related to
  insufficient knowledge of: (specify)
  Examples:
    Etiology
    Prevention
    Antibiotic
      prophylaxis

Signs and
  symptoms of
  complications

MYOCARDIAL INFARCTION
(Uncomplicated)

Collaborative Problems

Potential Complications:

Dysrhythmias
Cardiac arrest

Cardiogenic shock

Nursing Diagnoses

Pain related to cardiac tissue ischemia

Fear related to present status and unknown future

Sleep Pattern Disturbances related to treatments and environment

Potential Constipation related to bed rest, change in life-style, and medications

Activity Intolerance related to impaired oxygen transport secondary to decreased cardiac output and fear of recurrent angina

Potential Self-concept Disturbances related to perceived or actual role changes

Possible Impaired Home Maintenance Management related to angina or fear of angina

Potential Altered Family Processes related to impaired ability of ill person to assume role responsibilities

Potential Sexual Dysfunction related to fear of angina and altered self-concept

Grieving related to actual or perceived losses secondary to cardiac condition

Potential Altered Health Maintenance related to insufficient knowledge of: (specify)

Examples:

| Condition | Diet |
| Home activities | Medications |

Hematologic Conditions

ANEMIA

Collaborative Problems

Potential Complications:

| Transfusion reaction | Iron overload (repeated |
| Cardiac failure | transfusion) |

Nursing Diagnoses

Activity Intolerance related to impaired oxygen transport secondary to diminished red blood cell count

Potential for Infection related to decreased resistance secondary to tissue hypoxia and/

or abnormal white blood cells (neutropenia, leukopenia)

Potential for Injury: Bleeding Tendencies related to thrombocytopenia and splenomegaly

Potential Altered Oral Mucous Membrane related to gastrointestinal mucosal atrophy

Potential Altered Health Maintenance related to insufficient knowledge of: (specify)
Examples:

Condition	Drug therapy
Nutritional requirement	

APLASTIC ANEMIA

Collaborative Problems

Potential Complications:

Fatal aplasia	Hypoxia
Pancytopenia	Sepsis
Hemorrhage	

Nursing Diagnoses

Activity Intolerance related to insufficient oxygen secondary to diminished red blood cell count

Potential for Infection related to increased susceptibility secondary to leukopenia

Potential Altered Oral Mucous Membrane related to tissue hypoxia and vulnerability

Potential Altered Health Maintenance related to insufficient knowledge of: (specify)
Examples:

Causes	Signs and symptoms of complications
Prevention	

PERNICIOUS ANEMIA

See also Anemia.

Nursing Diagnoses

Altered Oral Mucous Membrane related to sore red tongue secondary to papillary atrophy and inflammatory changes

Diarrhea/Constipation related to gastrointestinal
mucosal atrophy
Potential Altered Nutrition: Less Than Body
Requirements related to anorexia secondary
to sore mouth
Potential Altered Health Maintenance related to
insufficient knowledge of: (specify)
Examples:

Chronicity of	Familial
disease	propensity
Vitamin B	
treatment	

DISSEMINATED INTRAVASCULAR COAGULATION (DIC)

See also Underlying Disorders (e.g., Obstetric, Infections, Burns).
See also Anticoagulant Therapy.

Collaborative Problems

Potential Complications:

Hemorrhage	Microthrombi (renal,
Renal failure	cardiac, pulmonary,
	cerebral,
	gastrointestinal)

Nursing Diagnoses

Fear related to treatments, environment, and
risk of death
Altered Family Processes related to critical
nature of the situation and uncertain
prognosis
Potential Sensory Perceptual Alterations
related to
Examples:
Pain
Immobility
Excessive environmental stimuli
Disruption of biorhythms
Potential Altered Health Maintenance related to
insufficient knowledge of: (specify)
Examples:

| Causes | Treatment |

POLYCYTHEMIA VERA

Collaborative Problems

Potential Complications:

Thrombus formation
Hemorrhage
Hypertension

Congestive heart
    failure
Peptic ulcer
Gout

Nursing Diagnoses

Altered Nutrition: Less Than Body
    Requirements related to anorexia, nausea,
    and vasocongestion
Activity Intolerance related to insufficient
    oxygenation secondary to pulmonary
    congestion and tissue hypoxia
Potential for Infection related to hypoxia
    secondary to vasocongestion
Potential Altered Health Maintenance related to
    insufficient knowledge of: (specify)
    Examples:
        Fluid requirements
        Exercise program
        Signs and symptoms of complications
            Thrombi
            Congestive heart failure
            Hypertension

Peripheral Vascular Conditions

DEEP VEIN THROMBOSIS

See also Anticoagulant Therapy, if indicated.

Collaborative Problems

Potential Complications:

Embolism
Chronic leg edema
Chronic stasis ulcers

Nursing Diagnoses

Potential Colonic Constipation related to
    immobility

Potential Altered Respiratory Function related to
    immobility

Potential Impaired Skin Integrity related to
    chronic ankle edema

Acute Pain related to impaired circulation
    (extremities)

Potential Altered Health Maintenance related to
    insufficient knowledge of: (specify)

  Examples:
    Prevention of recurrence
    Implications of anticoagulant therapy
    Exercise program
    Prevention of sequelae

HYPERTENSION

Collaborative Problems

Potential Complications:

Retinal hemorrhage   *Cerebral hemorrhage*
Cerebrovascular   *Renal failure*
    accident (CVA)

Nursing Diagnoses

Potential Noncompliance related to negative
    side-effects of prescribed therapy versus the
    belief that no treatment is needed without
    the presence of symptoms

Potential Sexual Dysfunction related to
    decreased libido or erectile dysfunction
    secondary to medication side-effects

Potential Altered Health Maintenance related to
    insufficient knowledge of: (specify)

  Examples:
    Diet restriction   Risk factors
    Medications   (obesity,
    Signs of   smoking)
      complications Follow-up care
                 Stress reduction
                 activities

VARICOSE VEINS

Collaborative Problems

Potential Complication: Vascular rupture
Potential Complication: Hemorrhage

Nursing Diagnoses

Chronic Pain related to engorgement of veins
Potential Altered Health Maintenance related to
    insufficient knowledge of: (specify)
    Examples:
        Condition
        Treatment options
        Risk factors

PERIPHERAL VASCULAR DISEASE
(Atherosclerosis, Arteriosclerosis)

Collaborative Problems

Potential Complications:

Stroke (CVA)
Ischemic ulcers
Claudication
Acute arterial thrombosis
Arterial embolization
Hypertension

Nursing Diagnoses

Altered Tissue Perfusion: Peripheral related to
    compromised circulation
Potential Impaired Tissue Integrity related to
    compromised circulation
Chronic Pain related to muscle ischemia during
    prolonged activity
Potential for Injury related to decreased
    sensation secondary to chronic
    atherosclerosis
Potential for Infection related to compromised
    circulation
Potential for Injury related to effects of
    orthostatic hypotension
Activity Intolerance related to claudication

Potential Altered Health Maintenance related to
insufficient knowledge of: (specify)
Examples:
Condition
Risk factors
Obesity
Cold
Signs and
symptoms of
complications

Prevention of
complications
Exercise program
Foot care
Smoking
Diet

RAYNAUD'S DISEASE/RAYNAUD'S SYNDROME

Collaborative Problems

Potential Complications:

Acute arterial occlusion
Ischemic ulcers
Gangrene

Nursing Diagnoses

Acute Pain related to ischemia secondary to
acute vasospasm
Altered Tissue Perfusion related to cold
environment
Potential Impaired Tissue Integrity: Ischemic
Ulcers related to vasospasm
Fear related to potential loss of work secondary
to condition
Potential Altered Health Maintenance related to
insufficient knowledge of: (specify)
Examples:
Condition
Stress
Cold
Stress reduction
techniques

Risk factors
Smoking
Vibrations

STASIS ULCERS (Postphlebitis Syndrome)

Collaborative Problems

Potential Complication: Cellulitis

Nursing Diagnoses

Altered Peripheral Tissue Perfusion related to
dependent position of legs
Potential for Infection related to compromised
circulation
Self-concept Disturbance related to chronic open
wounds
Chronic Pain related to ulcers and treatments
Potential Altered Health Maintenance related to
insufficient knowledge of: (specify)
Examples:
Etiology of ulcers
Risk factors
Prevention of injury, infection
Exercise program
Dressings
Need for compression

Respiratory Disorders

ADULT RESPIRATORY DISTRESS SYNDROME (ARDS)

*See also Mechanical Ventilation (under Diagnostic
Studies/Special Therapies).*

Collaborative Problems

Potential Complications:

Electrolyte imbalance   *Hypoxia*
*Of corticosteroid
therapy*

Nursing Diagnoses

Anxiety related to implications of condition and
critical care setting
Powerlessness related to condition and
treatments (ventilator, monitoring)

CHRONIC OBSTRUCTIVE PULMONARY DISEASE—COPD (Emphysema, Bronchitis)

Collaborative Problems

Potential Complications of Hypoxemia/ Hypovolemia:

Electrolyte imbalance
Acid–base imbalance

Inadequate cardiac
output

Nursing Diagnoses

Ineffective Airway Clearance related to excessive and tenacious mucus secretions

Altered Nutrition: Less Than Body Requirements related to dyspnea and anorexia

Activity Intolerance related to insufficient oxygenation for activities of daily living (ADL)

Impaired Verbal Communication related to dyspnea

Anxiety related to breathlessness and fear of suffocation

Powerlessness related to loss of control and the restrictions that this condition places on life-style

Sleep Pattern Disturbance related to
Examples:
Cough
Inability to assume recumbent position
Environment stimuli

Potential Altered Health Maintenance related to insufficient knowledge of: (specify)
Examples:
Condition
Pharmacologic
therapy
Nutritional
therapy
Prevention of
inflection

Rest versus
activity
Breathing
exercises
Home care (*e.g.*
equipment)

PLEURAL EFFUSION

See also Underlying Disorders (congestive heart disease, cirrhosis, malignancy).

Collaborative Problems

Potential Complications:

Respiratory failure Hypoxia
Pneumothorax (post- Hemothorax
   thoracentesis)

Nursing Diagnoses

Activity Intolerance related to insufficient
   oxygenation for ADL
Potential Altered Nutrition: Less Than Body
   Requirements related to anorexia secondary
   to pressure on abdominal structures
Altered Comfort: Pain and Dyspnea related to
   accumulation of fluid in pleural space
(Specify) Self-care Deficits related to fatigue and
   dyspnea

PNEUMONIA

Collaborative Problems

Potential Complications:

Hyperthermia Septic shock
Respiratory Paralytic ileus
   insufficiency

Nursing Diagnoses

Potential Altered Body Temperature related to
   infectious process
Activity Intolerance related to insufficient
   oxygenation for ADL
Potential Altered Oral Mucous Membrane
   related to mouth breathing and frequent
   expectorations
Potential Fluid Volume Deficit related to
   increased insensible fluid loss secondary to
   fever and hyperventilation

Potential Altered Nutrition: Less Than Body
Requirements related to anorexia, dyspnea,
and abdominal distention secondary to air
swallowing

Ineffective Airway Clearance related to pain,
tracheobronchial secretions, and exudate

Potential for Infection Transmission related to
communicable nature of the disease

Altered Comfort related to hyperthermia,
malaise, secondary to pulmonary pathology

Potential Impaired Skin Integrity related to
prescribed bed rest

Potential Altered Health Maintenance related to
insufficient knowledge of: (specify)

Examples:

Fluid requirements	Signs and symptoms of recurrence
Caloric requirements	Prevention of recurrence
Spread of infection	Medication regimen

PULMONARY EMBOLISM

Collaborative Problems

Potential Complication: Anticoagulant therapy
Potential Complication: Hypoxia

Nursing Diagnoses

Potential Impaired Skin Integrity related to
immobility and prescribed bed rest

Potential Altered Health Maintenance related to
insufficient knowledge of: (specify)

Examples:

Anticoagulant therapy	Signs and symptoms of complications

Metabolic/Endocrine Disorders

ADDISON'S DISEASE

Collaborative Problems

Potential Complications:

Addisonian crisis (shock) Hypoglycemia

Electrolyte imbalances (sodium, potassium)

Nursing Diagnoses

Potential Altered Nutrition: Less Than Body Requirements related to anorexia and nausea

Potential Fluid Volume Deficit related to excessive loss of sodium and water secondary to polyuria

Diarrhea related to increased excretion of sodium and water

Potential Self-concept Disturbance related to appearance changes secondary to increased skin pigmentation and decreased axillary and pubic hair (female)

Potential for Injury related to postural hypotension secondary to fluid/electrolyte imbalances

Potential Altered Health Maintenance related to insufficient knowledge of: (specify)

Examples:

Disease

Signs and symptoms of complications

Risks for crisis

Infection

Diarrhea

Decreased sodium intake

Diaphoresis

Overexertion

Dietary management

Identification (card, medallion)

Emergency kit

Pharmacologic management and titration
dose as needed

ALDOSTERONISM, PRIMARY

Collaborative Problems

Potential Complications:

Hypokalemia   Hypertension
Alkalosis   Hypernatremia

Nursing Diagnoses

Altered Comfort: Polydipsia related to excessive
   urine excretion
Potential Fluid Volume Deficit related to
   excessive urinary excretion
Potential Altered Health Maintenance related to
   insufficient knowledge of: (specify)
   Examples:
      Condition
      Surgical treatment
      Corticosteroid therapy

CIRRHOSIS (Laënnec's Disease)

See also Substance Abuse, if indicated.

Collaborative Problems

Potential Complications:

Hemorrhage   Drug toxicity (opiates,
Hypokalemia   short-acting
Portal systemic   barbiturates, major
   encephalopathy   tranquilizers)
Negative nitrogen   Renal failure
   balance   Anemia
                     Esophageal varices

Nursing Diagnoses

Chronic Pain related to liver enlargement and
   ascites
Diarrhea related to excessive secretion of fats in
   stool secondary to liver dysfunction

Potential for Injury related to decreased
prothrombin production and synthesis of
substances used in blood coagulation
Altered Nutrition: Less Than Body
Requirements related to anorexia, impaired
utilization, and storage of vitamins (A, C,
K, D, E)
Potential Altered Respiratory Function related to
pressure on diaphragm secondary to ascites
Potential Self-concept Disturbance related to
appearance changes (jaundice, ascites)
Potential for Infection related to leukopenia
secondary to enlarged, overactive spleen and
hypoproteinemia
Pruritus related to accumulation of bilirubin
pigment and bile salts
Fluid Volume Excess: Peripheral Edema related
to portal hypertension, lowered plasma
colloidal osmotic pressure, and sodium
retention
Potential Altered Health Maintenance related to
insufficient knowledge of: (specify)
Examples:
Pharmacologic contraindication
Nutritional requirements
Signs and symptoms of complications
Risks of alcohol ingestion

CUSHING'S SYNDROME

Collaborative Problems

Potential Complications:

Hypertension	*Psychosis*
Congestive heart	*Electrolyte imbalance*
failure	*(sodium, potassium)*

Nursing Diagnoses

Self-concept Disturbance related to physical
changes secondary to disease process (moon
face, thinning of hair, truncal obesity,
virilism)

Potential for Infection related to excessive
protein catabolism and depressed leukocytic
phagocytosis secondary to hyperglycemia

Potential for Injury: Fractures related to
osteoporosis

Potential Impaired Skin Integrity related to loss
of tissue, edema, and dryness

Altered Sexuality Patterns related to loss of
libido and cessation of menses (female)
secondary to excessive adrenocorticotropic
hormone production

Potential Altered Health Maintenance related to
insufficient knowledge of: (specify)
Examples:
Disease
Diet therapy
High protein
Low cholesterol
Low sodium

DIABETES MELLITUS

Collaborative Problems

Potential Complications:

Acute complications:
Ketoacidosis (DKA)
*Hyperosmolar hyperglycemic nonketotic coma
(HHNK)*
Hypoglycemia
Infections
Chronic complications:
Macrovascular
Cardiac artery disease (CAD)
Peripheral vascular disease (PVD)
Microvascular
Retinopathy
Neuropathy
Nephropathy
Mixed vascular and neuropathic complications
Leg and foot ulcer
Amputations

Nursing Diagnoses

Altered Health Maintenance related to deficient self-care practices

Potential for Injury related to decreased tactile sensation, diminished visual acuity, and hypoglycemia

Altered Comfort related to insulin injections, capillary blood glucose (CBG) testing, and diabetic peripheral neuropathy

Anxiety/Fear (individual, family) related to diagnosis of diabetes, potential complications of diabetes, and self-care regimens

Potential Ineffective Coping (individual, family) related to chronic disease, complex self-care regimen, and decreased support systems

Altered Nutrition: Greater Than Body Requirements related to intake in excess of need, lack of knowledge, and ineffective coping

Potential Sexual Dysfunction (male) related to peripheral neuropathy and/or psychological problems

Potential Sexual Dysfunction (female) related to physical and psychological stressors of diabetes

Powerlessness related to complications of diabetes (blindness, amputations, kidney failure, neuropathy)

Social Isolation related to visual impairment/blindness

Potential Noncompliance related to the complexity and chronicity of the prescribed regimen

Potential Altered Health Maintenance related to insufficient knowledge of: (specify)
  Examples:
    ADA exchange diet
    Weight control
    Weight maintenance
    Benefits/risks of exercise
    Self-monitoring of blood glucose (SMBG)
    Medications

Sick day care
Foot care
Hypoglycemia
Available resources

HEPATITIS (Acute, Viral)

Collaborative Problems

Potential Complications:

Hepatic failure
Coma

Subacute hepatic
necrosis
Fulminant hepatitis

Nursing Diagnoses

Fatigue related to weakness secondary to
reduced energy metabolism by liver
Potential for Infection Transmission related to
contagious agents
Altered Nutrition: Less Than Body
Requirements related to anorexia, epigastric
distress, and nausea
Potential Fluid Volume Deficit related to lack of
desire to drink
Pruritus related to bile salt accumulation
Potential for Injury related to reduced
prothrombin synthesis and reduced vitamin
K absorption
Altered Comfort related to swelling of inflamed
liver
Diversional Activity Deficit related to the
monotony of confinement and isolation
precautions
Potential Altered Health Maintenance related to
insufficient knowledge of: (specify)
  Examples:
    Condition
    Rest requirements
    Precautions to prevent transmission
    Nutritional requirements
    Contraindications
      Certain medications
      Alcohol

HYPERTHYROIDISM

(Thyrotoxicosis, Graves' Disease)

Collaborative Problems

Potential Complication: *Thyroid storm*
Potential Complication: *Cardiac dysrhythmias*

Nursing Diagnoses

Altered Nutrition: Less Than Body
    Requirements related to intake less than
    metabolic needs secondary to excessive
    metabolic rate

Activity Intolerance related to fatigue and
    exhaustion secondary to excessive metabolic
    rate

Diarrhea related to increased peristalsis
    secondary to excessive metabolic rate

Altered Comfort related to heat intolerance and
    profuse diaphoresis

Potential Impaired Tissue Integrity: Corneal
    related to inability to close eyelids
    secondary to exophthalmos

Potential for Injury related to tremors

Potential Hyperthermia related to lack of
    metabolic compensatory mechanism
    secondary to hyperthyroidism

Potential Altered Health Maintenance related to
    insufficient knowledge of: (specify)
    Examples:
        Condition
        Treatment regimen
        Pharmacologic therapy
        Eye care
        Dietary management
        Signs and symptoms of complications

HYPOTHYROIDISM (Myxedema)

Collaborative Problems

Potential Complications:

Atherosclerotic heart disease	*Acute organic psychosis*
Normochromic, normocytic anemia	*Myxedemic coma*

Nursing Diagnoses

Altered Nutrition: More Than Body
Requirements related to intake greater than
metabolic needs secondary to slowed
metabolic rate

Activity Intolerance related to insufficient
oxygenation secondary to slowed metabolic
rate

Colonic Constipation related to decreased
peristaltic action secondary to decreased
metabolic rate and decreased physical
activity

Impaired Skin Integrity related to edema and
dryness secondary to decreased metabolic
rate and infiltration of fluid into interstitial
tissues

Altered Comfort related to cold intolerance
secondary to decreased metabolic rate

Potential Impaired Social Interactions related to
listlessness and depression

Impaired Verbal Communication related to
slowed speech secondary to enlarged tongue

Potential Altered Health Maintenance related to
insufficient knowledge of: (specify)

Examples:

Condition	Pharmacologic
Treatment	therapy
regimen	Sensitivity to
Dietary	narcotics,
management	barbiturates,
Signs and	and
symptoms of	anesthetic
complications	agents

OBESITY

Nursing Diagnoses

Altered Health Maintenance related to
imbalance between caloric intake and
energy expenditure

Ineffective Individual Coping related to increase
in food consumption as a response to
stressors

Chronic Low Self-esteem related to feelings of
self-degradation and the response of others
to the condition

PANCREATITIS

Collaborative Problems

Potential Complications:

Shock
Hemorrhagic
  pancreatitis
Respiratory failure

Pleural effusion
Hypocalcemia
Hyperglycemia

Nursing Diagnoses

Pain related to nasogastric suction, distention of
pancreatic capsule, and local peritonitis
Potential Fluid Volume Deficit related to
decreased intake secondary to nausea and
vomiting
Altered Nutrition: Less Than Body
Requirements related to vomiting and diet
restrictions
Diarrhea related to excessive excretion of fats in
stools secondary to insufficient pancreatic
enzymes
Potential Altered Health Maintenance related to
insufficient knowledge of: (specify)
Examples:
Disease
Contraindications
Alcohol
Coffee
Large meals
Dietary management
Follow-up care

Gastrointestinal Disorders

ESOPHAGEAL DISORDERS (Esophagitis, Hiatal Hernia)

Collaborative Problems

Potential Complication: Hemorrhage
Potential Complication: Gastric ulcers

Nursing Diagnoses

Potential Altered Nutrition: Less Than Body
  Requirements related to anorexia,
  heartburn, and dysphagia
Altered Comfort: Heartburn related to
  regurgitation and eructation
Potential Altered Health Maintenance related to
  insufficient knowledge of: (specify)
  Examples:

Condition	Positioning after
Dietary	meals
management	Pharmacologic
Hazards of	therapy
alcohol and	Weight reduction
tobacco	(if indicated)

GASTROENTERITIS

Nursing Diagnoses

Potential Fluid Volume Deficit related to
  vomiting and diarrhea
Altered Comfort related to abdominal cramps,
  diarrhea, and vomiting
Potential Altered Health Maintenance related to
  insufficient knowledge of: (specify)
  Examples:

Condition	Signs and
Dietary	symptoms of
restrictions	complications

HEMORRHOIDS/ANAL FISSURE

(Nonsurgical)

Collaborative Problems

Potential Complications:

Bleeding	Thrombosis
Strangulation	

Nursing Diagnoses

Altered Comfort related to pain on defecation

Potential Altered Bowel Elimination:
  Constipation related to fear of pain on defecation

Potential Altered Health Maintenance related to insufficient knowledge of: (specify)
  Examples:
  Condition   Exercise program
  Bowel routine   Perianal care
  Diet instructions

INFLAMMATORY INTESTINAL DISORDERS (Diverticulosis, Diverticulitis, Regional Enteritis, Ulcerative Colitis)

Collaborative Problems

Potential Complications:

Anal fissure   Anemia
Perianal abscess,   Intestinal obstruction
  fissure, fistula
Fluid/electrolyte
  imbalances

Nursing Diagnoses

Altered Comfort related to intestinal inflammatory process

Diarrhea related to intestinal inflammatory process

Colonic Constipation related to inadequate dietary intake of fiber

Potential Impaired Skin Integrity (Perianal) related to diarrhea and chemical irritants

Potential Ineffective Individual Coping related to the chronicity of the condition and the lack of definitive treatment

Altered Nutrition: Less Than Body Requirements related to diarrhea, dietary restrictions, and pain with or after eating and/or painful ulcers in the mouth

Altered Health Maintenance related to
inadequate stress management and exercise
program
Potential Altered Health Maintenance related to
insufficient knowledge of: (specify)
Examples:

Condition	Signs and
Dietary	symptoms of
restrictions	complications
Treatment	

PEPTIC ULCER

Collaborative Problems

Potential Complications:

Hemorrhage	Pyloric obstruction
Perforation	

Nursing Diagnoses

Altered Comfort related to lesions secondary to
increased gastric secretions
Potential Colonic Constipation related to diet
restrictions and side-effects of medications
Potential Altered Health Maintenance related to
insufficient knowledge of: (specify)
Examples:
Condition
Dietary restrictions
Contraindications

Certain	Tobacco
medications	Caffeine
Alcohol	

Signs and symptoms of complications

Renal/Urinary Tract Disorders

NEUROGENIC BLADDER

Collaborative Problems

Potential Complication: *Renal calculi*
Potential Complication: *Autonomic dysreflexia*

Nursing Diagnoses

Potential Impaired Skin Integrity related to
constant irritation from urine

Potential for Infection related to retention of
urine and/or introduction of urinary
catheter

Potential Social Isolation related to
embarrassment from wetting oneself in
front of others and fear of offending others
with odor from urine

Urinary Retention related to chronically
overfilled bladder with loss of sensation of
bladder distention

Reflex Incontinence related to absence of
sensation to void and loss of ability to
inhibit bladder contraction

Potential Altered Health Maintenance related to
insufficient knowledge of: (specify)
Examples:
Etiology
Treatment/bladder retraining programs
Signs and symptoms of complications
Prevention of complications

RENAL FAILURE (Acute)

Collaborative Problems

Potential Complications:

Fluid overload	*Hyperkalemia*
Hyperphosphatemia	*Metabolic acidosis*

Nursing Diagnoses

Altered Nutrition: Less Than Body
Requirements related to anorexia, dietary
restrictions, and altered taste

Potential for Infection related to invasive
procedures

Anxiety related to present status and unknown
prognosis

RENAL FAILURE (Chronic, Uremia)

*See also Peritoneal Dialysis and Hemodialysis, if
indicated.*

Collaborative Problems

Potential Complications:

Fluid/electrolyte
  imbalance
Hypertension
Gastrointestinal
  bleeding
Hyperparathyroidism
Pathological fractures
Malnutrition
Anemia,
  thrombocytopenia

Hypoalbuminemia
Polyneuropathy
  (peripheral)
Congestive heart
  failure
Pulmonary edema
Metabolic acidosis
Pleural effusion
Pericarditis

Nursing Diagnoses

Fluid Volume Excess: Peripheral Edema related
    to fluid and electrolyte imbalances
    secondary to renal dysfunction
Altered Nutrition: Less Than Body
    Requirements related to
  Examples:
    Anorexia   Stomatitis
    Nausea/vomiting   Unpalatable diet
    Loss of taste,
      smell
Sexual Dysfunction or Altered Sexuality Patterns
    related to
  Examples:
    Decreased libido   Amenorrhea
    Impotence   Sterility
Self-concept Disturbance related to effects of
    limitation on achievement of developmental
    tasks
Potential Social Isolation (Individual, Family)
    related to disability and treatment
    requirements
Altered Comfort related to
  Examples:
    Fatigue   Fluid retention
    Headaches   Anemia
Fatigue related to insufficient oxygenation
    secondary to anemia
Pruritus related to abnormal deposition of
    calcium secondary to calcium/phosphate
    imbalance

Powerlessness related to progessively disabling
nature of disorder
Potential Altered Health Maintenance related to
insufficient knowledge of: (specify)
Examples:
Condition
Fluid and sodium restrictions
Dietary restrictions
Protein
Potassium
Sodium
Daily recording
Intake
Output
Weights
Pharmacologic therapy
Signs/symptoms of complications
Follow-up visits
Community resources (support groups)

URINARY TRACT INFECTIONS
(Cystitis, Pyelonephritis, Glomerulonephritis)
See also Acute Renal Failure.

Nursing Diagnoses
Chronic Pain related to inflammation and tissue
trauma
Altered Comfort: Dysuria related to
inflammation and infection
Potential Altered Nutrition: Less Than Body
Requirements related to anorexia secondary
to malaise
Potential Ineffective Individual Coping related to
the chronicity of the condition
Potential Altered Health Maintenance related to
insufficient knowledge of: (specify)
Examples:
Prevention of recurrence
Adequate fluid intake
Frequent voiding
Hygiene measures (personal, post-
toileting)
Voiding after sexual activity
Signs/symptoms of recurrence
Pharmacologic therapy

UROLITHIASIS (Renal Calculi)

Collaborative Problems

Potential Complication: Pyelonephritis
Potential Complication: Acute renal failure

Nursing Diagnoses

Altered Comfort related to inflammation
    secondary to irritation of stone
Diarrhea related to renointestinal reflexes
Potential Altered Health Maintenance related to
    insufficient knowledge of: (specify)
    Examples:
        Prevention of recurrence
        Dietary restrictions
        Fluid requirements

Neurologic Disorders

BRAIN TUMOR

*Because this disorder can cause alterations varying
    from minimal to profound, the following possible
    nursing diagnoses reflect individuals with varying
    degrees of involvement.*
See also Surgery (General, Cranial).
See also Cancer.

Collaborative Problems

Potential Complications:
    Increased intracranial   Motor losses
        pressure   Sensory losses
    Paralysis   Cognitive losses
    Hyperthermia

Nursing Diagnoses

Potential for Injury related to gait disorders,
    vertigo and/or visual disturbances,
    compression/displacement of brain tissue
Anxiety related to implications of condition and
    uncertain future

(Specify) Self-care Deficit related to inability to
perform/difficulty in performing activities of
daily living secondary to sensory-motor
impairments

Altered Nutrition: Less Than Body
Requirements related to dysphagia and
fatigue

Grieving related to actual/perceived loss of
function and uncertain future

Impaired Physical Mobility related to sensory-
motor impairment

Altered Comfort: Headache related to
compression/displacement of brain tissue
and increased intracranial pressure

Altered Family Processes related to the nature of
the condition, role disturbances, and
uncertain future

Self-concept Disturbance related to interruption
in achieving/failure to achieve
developmental tasks (childhood,
adolescence, young adulthood, middle age)

Potential Fluid Volume Deficit related to
vomiting secondary to increased intracranial
pressure

Potential for Injury related to impaired/
uncontrolled sensory-motor function

CEREBROVASCULAR ACCIDENT

*Because this disorder can cause alterations varying
from minimal to profound, the following possible
nursing diagnoses reflect individuals with varying
degrees of involvement.*

Collaborative Problems

Potential Complications:

Increased intracranial pressure
Pneumonia
Atelectasis

Nursing Diagnoses

Sensory–Perceptual Alterations: (specify) related
to hypoxia and compression or
displacement of brain tissue

Impaired Verbal Communication related to
dysarthria and/or aphasia

Potential for Injury related to

Examples:

Visual field deficits	Inability to perceive environmental hazards
Motor deficits	
Perception deficits	

Activity Intolerance related to

Examples:

Fatigue	Inability to tolerate increased activity
Weakness	

Potential For Disuse Syndrome related to effects
of immobility

(Specify type) Incontinence related to

Examples:

Loss of bladder tone

Loss of sphincter control

Inability to perceive bladder cues

(Specify) Self-care Deficit related to (specify)

Impaired Swallowing related to (specify)

Grieving (Family, Individual) related to actual or
perceived loss of function and inability to
meet role responsibilities

Potential Impaired Social Interactions related to
difficulty communicating and
embarrassment regarding disabilities

Potential Fluid Volume Deficit related to

Examples:

Dysphagia	Fatigue
Difficulty in obtaining fluids	Weakness
	Sensory-motor deficits

Potential Impaired Home Maintenance
Management related to altered ability to
maintain self at home secondary to sensory-
motor/cognitive deficits

Unilateral Neglect related to (specify site)
secondary to effects of cerebral pathology

Potential Altered Health Maintenance related to
insufficient knowledge of: (specify)

Examples:

Condition

Pharmacologic therapy

Self-care activities of daily living
Home care
Speech therapy
Exercise program
Community resources
Self-help groups
Signs and symptoms of complications
Skin care
Bowel/bladder program
Reality orientation
Possible behavioral responses
Lability
Regression

NERVOUS SYSTEM DISORDERS

(Degenerative, Demyelinating, Inflammatory;
Myasthenia Gravis, Multiple Sclerosis,
Muscular Dystrophy, Parkinson's Disease,
Guillain-Barré Syndrome, Amyotrophic
Lateral Sclerosis)

*Because the alterations associated with these
disorders can range from minimal to profound,
the following possible nursing diagnoses reflect
individuals with varying degrees of involvement.*

Collaborative Problems

Potential Complications:

Renal failure   Atelectasis
Pneumonia

Nursing Diagnoses

Self-concept Disturbance related to prolonged
debilitating condition and interruption in
achieving development tasks (adolescence,
young adulthood, middle age)
Potential for Injury related to
Examples:
Visual   Weakness
  disturbances   Uncontrolled
Unsteady gait   movements
Impaired Verbal Communication related to
dysarthrias secondary to cranial nerve
impairment

Potential Altered Nutrition: Less Than Body Requirements related to dysphagia/chewing difficulties secondary to cranial nerve impairment

Activity Intolerance related to fatigue and difficulty in performing activities of daily living

Potential For Disuse Syndrome related to effects of immobility

Urinary Retention related to sensory-motor deficits

Grieving (Patient, Family) related to nature of disease and uncertain prognosis

Altered Sexuality Pattern (Female) related to loss of libido, fatigue, and decreased perineal sensation

Sexual Dysfunction (Male): Impotence related to neurosensory deficits

Potential for Injury related to decreased perception of pain, touch, and temperature

Altered Family Processes related to nature of disease, role disturbances, and uncertain future

Potential Diversional Activity Deficits related to inability to perform usual job-related/ recreational activities

Potential Social Isolation related to mobility difficulties and associated embarrassment

Impaired Home Maintenance Management related to inability to care for/difficulty in caring for self/home secondary to disability or unavailable or inadequate caregiver

Parental Role Conflict related to disruptions secondary to disability

Ineffective Individual Coping related to implications of disease and its prognosis

(Specify) Self-care Deficits related to
Examples:
Headaches	Fatigue
Muscular spasms	Paresis/paralysis
Joint pain	

Powerlessness related to inability to control symptoms and the unpredictable nature of the condition (*i.e.,* remissions/ exacerbations)

Incontinence: (specify type) related to (specify)

Ineffective Airway Clearance related to impaired
    ability to cough
Potential Altered Health Maintenance related to
    insufficient knowledge of: (specify)
    Examples:
        Condition
        Risks
            Severe fatigue
            Infection
            Cold
            Fever
            Pregnancy
        Exercise program
        Nutritional requirements
        Community services
        Medications
            Schedule
            Side-effects

PRESENILE DEMENTIA (Alzheimer's Disease, Huntington's Disease)

*See also Nervous System Diseases.**

Nursing Diagnoses

Potential for Injury related to lack of awareness
    of environmental hazard
Altered Thought Processes related to an inability
    to evaluate reality secondary to cerebral
    neuron degeneration
Impaired Physical Mobility related to gait
    instability
Potential Altered Family Processes related to
    effects of condition on relationships, role
    responsibilities, and finances
Impaired Home Maintenance Management
    related to inability to care for/difficulty in
    caring for self/home or inadequate/
    unavailable caregiver

* Because these disorders can cause alterations similar to
those in the nervous system disorder category, the reader is
referred to the latter section to review additional possible
diagnoses.

Unilateral Neglect related to (specify site)
secondary to neurological pathology
(Specify) Self-care Deficit related to (specify)
Decisional Conflict related to placement of
person in a care facility

SEIZURE DISORDERS (Epilepsy)

*If the client is a child, see also Development
Problems/Needs.*

Nursing Diagnoses

Potential for Injury related to uncontrolled
tonic/clonic movements during seizure
episode
Potential Social Isolation related to fear of a
seizure in public (embarrassment)
Potential Altered Growth and Development
related to interruption in achieving/failure
to achieve developmental tasks (childhood,
adolescence, young adulthood, middle age)
Potential Altered Oral Mucous Membrane
related to effects of drug therapy on oral
tissue
Fear related to unpredictable nature of seizures
and embarrassment
Potential Altered Health Maintenance related to
insufficient knowledge of: (specify)
Examples:
Condition
Medication
Schedule
Side-effects
Activity versus rest (balance)
Care during seizure
Community resources
Possible environmental hazards
Swimming
Diving
Operating machinery
Identification
Medallion
Card

SPINAL CORD INJURY*

Collaborative Problems

Potential Complications:

Accidental extension
of injury (acute)
Autonomic dysreflexia
(postacute)
Electrolyte imbalance
Spinal shock
Hemorrhage
Respiratory
complications

Paralytic ileus
Sepsis
Neurogenic bladder
Hydronephrosis
Gastrointestinal
bleeding
Thrombophlebitis
(deep vein)
Postural hypotension

Nursing Diagnoses

(Specify) Self-care Deficit related to sensory-
motor deficits secondary to level of spinal
cord injury

Impaired Verbal Communication related to
impaired ability to speak words secondary
to tracheostomy

Fear related to
Examples:
Abandonment by others
Changes in role responsibilities
Effects of injury on life-style
Multiple tests and procedures
Separation from support systems

Grieving related to anticipated losses secondary
to sensory-motor deficits

Altered Family Processes related to adjustment
requirements for the situation (time, energy,
financial, physical care, prognosis)

Potential for Aspiration related to inability to
cough secondary to level of injury

Potential Impaired Home Maintenance
Management related to inadequate
resources, housing, or impaired caregiver(s)

---

* Because disabilities associated with spinal cord injuries
can be varied (hemiparesis, quadriparesis, diplegia, mono-
plegia, triplegia, paraplegia), the nurse will have to specify
clearly the individual's limitations in the diagnostic statement.

Potential Social Isolation (Individual/Family) related to disability or requirements for the caregiver(s)

Potential Altered Parenting related to inadequate resources and coping mechanisms

Self-concept Disturbance related to effects of limitations on achievement of developmental tasks

Potential Fluid Volume Deficit related to difficulty obtaining liquids

Potential Altered Nutrition: More Than Body Requirements related to imbalance of intake versus activity expenditures

Potential Altered Nutrition: Less Than Body Requirements related to anorexia and increased metabolic requirements

Potential Diversional Activity Deficit related to effects of limitations on ability to participate in recreational activities

Reflex Incontinence or Urinary Retention related to bladder atony secondary to sensory-motor deficits

Potential For Disuse Syndrome related to effects of immobility

Potential for Injury related to impaired ability to control movements and sensory-motor deficits

Potential for Infection related to
Examples:
Urinary stasis
Repeated catheterizations
Invasive procedures
Skeletal tongs
Tracheostomy
Venous lines
Surgical sites

Potential Sexual Dysfunction related to
Examples:
Inability to achieve or sustain an erection for intercourse
Limitations on sexual performance
Value conflicts regarding sexual expression
Depression/anxiety
Decreased libido
Altered self-concept
Unwilling/uninformed partner

Potential Altered Health Maintenance related to
insufficient knowledge of: (specify)
Examples:
Condition Rehabilitation
Treatment Assistance devices
regimen

UNCONSCIOUS INDIVIDUAL

See also Mechanical Ventilation, if indicated.

Collaborative Problems

Potential Complications:

Respiratory Bladder distention
insufficiency Seizures
Pneumonia Stress ulcers
Atelectasis Increased intracranial
Fluid/electrolyte pressure
imbalance
Negative nitrogen
balance

Nursing Diagnoses

Potential for Infection related to immobility and
invasive devices (tracheostomy, Foley
catheter, venous lines)
Potential Impaired Tissue Integrity: Corneal
related to corneal drying secondary to open
eyes and lower tear production
Anxiety/Fear (Family) related to present state of
individual and uncertain prognosis
Potential Altered Oral Mucous Membrane
related to inability to perform mouth care
on self and pooling of secretions
Total Self-care Deficit related to unconscious
state
Total Incontinence related to unconscious state
Potential For Disuse Syndrome related to effects
of immobility

Sensory Disorders

OPHTHALMIC DISORDERS (Cataracts, Detached Retina, Glaucoma, Inflammations)

See also Cataract Extractions
See also Scleral Buckle/Vitrectomy

Nursing Diagnoses

Potential for Injury related to impaired vision
secondary to condition or eye patches

Pain related to
Examples:
Inflammation
Lid
Lacrimal structures
Conjunctiva
Uveal tract
Retina
Cornea
Sclera
Infection
Increased intraocular pressure
Ocular tumors

Potential Noncompliance related to side-effects
of medications, difficulty remembering, and
financial impact

Potential Social Isolation related to fear of injury
or embarrassment outside home
environment

Potential Impaired Home Maintenance
Management related to impaired ability to
perform activities of daily living secondary
to impaired vision

(Specify) Self-care Deficit related to impaired
vision

Anxiety related to the actual or possible loss of
vision and/or surgical procedure

Potential Altered Health Maintenance related to
insufficient knowledge of: (specify)
Examples:
Condition
Eye care
Patches
Compresses
Medications
Eye drops
Instillation
Safety measures
Activity restrictions
Follow-up care

OTIC DISORDERS (Infections, Mastoiditis, Trauma)

Nursing Diagnoses

Potential for Injury related to disturbances of balance and impaired ability to detect environmental hazards

Impaired Verbal Communication related to difficulty understanding others secondary to impaired hearing

Potential Impaired Social Interactions related to difficulty in participating in conversations

Social Isolation related to the lack of contact with others secondary to fear and embarrassment of hearing losses

Pain related to
  Examples:
    Inflammation   Tinnitus
    Infection   Vertigo

Fear related to actual or possible loss of hearing

Potential Altered Health Maintenance related to insufficient knowledge of: (specify)
  Examples:
    Condition
    Medications
    Prevention of recurrence
    Hazards
      Swimming
      Air travel
      Showers
    Signs and symptoms of complications
    Hearing aids

Integumentary Disorders

DERMATOLOGIC DISORDERS (Dermatitis, Psoriasis, Eczema)

Nursing Diagnoses

Impaired Skin Integrity related to lesions and inflammatory response

Pruritus related to dermal eruptions

Potential Impaired Social Interaction related to fear of embarrassment and negative reactions of others

Potential Self-concept Disturbance related to
appearance and response of others
Potential Altered Health Maintenance related to
insufficient knowledge of: (specify)
Examples:
Condition   Contraindications
Topical agents

PRESSURE ULCERS*

Nursing Diagnoses

Potential for Infection related to susceptibility of
open wound
Impaired Tissue Integrity: Pressure Ulcers
related to
Examples:
Skin deficits (edema, obesity, dryness)
Impaired oxygen transport (edema,
peripheral anemia)
Chemical/mechanical irritants (casts,
radiation, incontinence)
Nutritional deficits
Systemic deficits (infection, cancer, renal or
hepatic disorders, diabetes mellitus)
Sensory deficits (confusion, cord injury,
neuropathy)
Immobility
Impaired Home Maintenance Management
related to complexity of care or unavailable
caregiver

The following are some situations that contribute
to pressure sore development. If the situation is pres-
ent in the client, the nursing diagnosis can be used.
Altered Nutrition: Less Than Body
Requirements related to anorexia secondary
to (specify)
Impaired Physical Mobility related to (specify)
Fluid Volume Excess: Edema related to (specify)
Total Incontinence related to (specify)

* The factors that can contribute to the development of
pressure sores are varied and complex; therefore, the nurse
must assess for and identify the specific etiologic/contributing
risk factors for the individual.

Sensory–Perceptual Alterations: Inability to Feel or Perceive Pressure related to (specify)

Potential Altered Health Maintenance related to insufficient knowledge of: (specify)

Examples:

Causes   Treatment
Preventive
    measures

SKIN INFECTIONS (Impetigo, Herpes Zoster, Fungal Infections)

Collaborative Problems

Potential Complications (Herpes Zoster):

Post-herpetic neuralgia   Corneal ulceration
Keratitis   Blindness
Uveitis

Nursing Diagnoses

Impaired Skin Integrity related to lesions and pruritus

Altered Comfort: Pain, Pruritus related to dermal eruptions

Potential for Infection Transmission related to contagious nature of the organism

Potential Altered Health Maintenance related to insufficient knowledge of: (specify)

Examples:

Condition (causes, course)
Prevention
Treatments
Skin care

THERMAL INJURIES (Burns, Severe Hypothermia)

Acute Period

Collaborative Problems

Potential Complications:

Death   Anemia
Fluid-loss shock   Negative nitrogen
Fluid overload   balance

Septicemia	Convulsive disorders
Emboli	Stress diabetes
Graft rejection	Adrenocortical
Hypothermia	insufficiency
Hypokalemia/	Pneumonia
hyperkalemia	Renal failure
Curling's ulcer	Compartmental
Paralytic ileus	syndrome

Nursing Diagnoses

Potential for Infection related to loss of
protective layer secondary to thermal injury

Altered Nutrition: Less Than Body
Requirements related to increased caloric
requirement secondary to thermal injury
and inability to ingest increased
requirements

Acute Pain related to thermal injury and
treatments

(Specify) Self-care Deficit related to impaired
range-of-motion ability secondary to pain
and contractures

Fear related to painful procedures and possibility
of death

Potential Social Isolation related to infection
control measures and separation from
family and support systems

Potential For Disuse Syndrome related to effects
of pain and immobility

Sleep Pattern Disturbances related to position
restrictions, pain, and treatment
interruptions

Potential Sensory–Perceptual Alterations
related to
Examples:

Excessive	Imposed
environmental	immobility
stimuli	Sleep deprivation
Stress	Protective
	isolation

Grieving (Family, Individual) related to actual or
perceived impact of injury on life
(appearance, relationships, occupation)

Postacute Period

If individual is a child, see also Developmental Problems/Needs.

Collaborative Problems

Potential Complications: Same as in acute period

Nursing Diagnoses

Diversional Activity Deficit related to monotony of confinement

Potential Social Isolation related to embarrassment and the response of others to injury

Powerlessness related to inability to control present situation

Self-concept Disturbance related to effects of thermal injury on achieving developmental tasks (child, adolescent, adult)

Fear related to uncertain future and effects of injury on life-style, relationships, occupation

Impaired Home Maintenance Management related to long-term requirements of treatments

Potential Altered Health Maintenance related to insufficient knowledge of: (specify)

    Examples:

        Condition

        Treatment

            Surgery

            Whirlpool

        Nutritional requirements

        Pain management

        Home care

        Rehabilitation

        Community services

Musculoskeletal/ Connective Tissue Disorders

FRACTURED JAW

Nursing Diagnoses

Potential for Aspiration related to inadequate cough secondary to pain and fixative devices

Altered Oral Mucous Membrane related to difficulty in performing oral hygiene secondary to fixation devices

Impaired Verbal Communication related to fixation devices

Acute Pain related to tissue trauma

Potential Altered Nutrition: Less Than Body Requirements related to inability to ingest solid food secondary to fixation devices

Potential Altered Health Maintenance related to insufficient knowledge of: (specify)
Examples:
Mouth care
Nutritional requirements
Signs and symptoms of infection
Procedure for emergency wire cutting (*e.g.,* vomiting)

FRACTURES

See also Casts.

Collaborative Problems

Potential Complications:

Neurovascular (paresis, paralysis)
Fat embolism syndrome
Shock (hemorrhagic, hypovolemic)
Misalignment
Osteomyelitis
Compartmental syndrome
Contracture

Nursing Diagnoses

Acute Pain related to tissue trauma

Potential Impaired Skin Integrity related to mechanical irritants/compression secondary to casts and traction

Potential For Disuse Syndrome related to effects of immobility secondary to casts/traction

Potential for Infection related to invasive fixation devices

(Specify) Self-care Deficits related to impaired ability to use upper/lower limb secondary to immobilization device

Diversional Activity Deficit related to boredom of confinement secondary to immobilization devices

Potential Impaired Home Maintenance Management related to

Examples:
Fixation device   Unavailable
Impaired physical   support
   mobility   system

Altered Family Processes related to difficulty of ill person in assuming role responsibilities secondary to limited motion

Potential Altered Health Maintenance related to insufficient knowledge of: (specify)

Examples:
Condition
Cast care
Use of assistive devices
   Cane
   Crutches
   Walker
Signs and symptoms of complications
   Numbness
   Pallor
   Decreased sensation
Limitations

LOW BACK PAIN

Collaborative Problems

Potential Complication: Herniated nucleus pulposus

Nursing Diagnoses

Pain related to
  Examples:
    Acute   Weak muscles
      lumbosacral   Osteoarthritis of
      strain   spine
    Unstable   Spinal stenosis
      lumbosacral   Intervertebral disk
      ligaments   problem
  Impaired Physical Mobility related to decreased
    mobility and flexibility secondary to muscle
    spasm
  Potential Ineffective Individual Coping:
    Depression related to effects of chronic pain
    on life-style
  Potential Altered Family Processes related to
    impaired ability to meet role responsibilities
    (financial, home, social)
  Potential Altered Health Maintenance related to
    insufficient knowledge of: (specify)
    Examples:
    Condition
    Exercise program
    Noninvasive pain relief methods
      Relaxation
      Imagery
    Proper posture and body mechanics

OSTEOMYELITIS

Collaborative Problems

Potential Complication: Bone abscess

Nursing Diagnoses

Pain related to soft tissue edema secondary to
  infection
Impaired Physical Mobility related to limited
  range of motion of affected bone
Potential Altered Health Maintenance related to
  insufficient knowledge of: (specify)
Examples
  Condition
    Etiology
    Course

Pharmacologic therapy
Nutritional requirements
Pain management
Signs and symptoms of complications

OSTEOPOROSIS

Collaborative Problems

Potential Complications:

Fractures   Paralytic ileus
Kyphosis

Nursing Diagnoses

Pain related to muscle spasm and fractures
Altered Health Maintenance related to
insufficient daily physical activity
Altered Nutrition: Less Than Body
Requirements related to inadequate dietary
intake of calcium, protein, and vitamin D
Impaired Physical Mobility related to limited
range of motion secondary to skeletal
changes
Fear related to unpredictable nature of condition
Potential for Injury: Fractures related to porous
bones secondary to disease process
Potential Altered Health Maintenance related to
insufficient knowledge of: (specify)
Examples:
Condition
Etiology
Course
Nutritional therapy
Activity program
Safety precautions
Prevention

INFLAMMATORY JOINT DISEASE

Nursing Diagnoses

Pain related to inflammatory response and joint
immobility (stiffness)
(Specify) Self-care Deficits related to loss of

motion, muscle weakness, pain, stiffness, or fatigue

Ineffective Individual Coping related to the stress imposed by exacerbations (unpredictable)

Self-concept Disturbance related to physical and psychological changes imposed by the disease

Fatigue related to effects of chronic inflammatory process

Potential Altered Oral Mucous Membrane related to medications and decreased saliva

Impaired Home Maintenance Management related to impaired ability to perform household responsibilities secondary to limited mobility

Sleep Pattern Disturbance related to pain and/or secondary to fibrositis

Impaired Physical Mobility related to pain and limited motion of limbs

Sexual Dysfunction related to difficulty assuming position (female), fatigue, pain, or decreased lubrication

Potential Social Isolation related to ambulation difficulties and fatigue

Altered Family Processes related to difficulty in assuming/inability to assume role responsibilities secondary to fatigue and limited motion

Potential Altered Health Maintenance related to insufficient knowledge of: (specify)

Examples:

Condition	Quackery
Rest vs. exercise	Heat therapy
Self-help groups	Pharmacologic
Assistive devices	therapy

Infectious/ Immunodeficient Disorders

LUPUS ERYTHEMATOSUS (Systemic)

See also Rheumatic Diseases.
See also Corticosteroid Therapy.

Collaborative Problems

Potential Complications:

Renal failure secondary to corticosteroid therapy
Pericarditis
Pleuritis

Nursing Diagnoses

Powerlessness related to unpredictable course
(remissions, exacerbations)
Ineffective Individual Coping related to
unpredictable course and altered appearance
Potential Social Isolation related to
embarrassment and the response of others
to appearance
Potential Self-concept Disturbance related to
inability to achieve developmental tasks
secondary to disabling condition
Potential Altered Health Maintenance related to
insufficient knowledge of: (specify)
Examples:

Condition	Pharmacologic
Rest/activity	therapy
balance	

MENINGITIS/ENCEPHALITIS

Collaborative Problems

Potential Complications:

Fluid/electrolyte	*Seizures*
imbalance	*Septicemia*
Cerebral edema	*Alkalosis*
Adrenal damage	*Increased intracranial*
Circulatory collapse	*pressure*
Hemorrhage	

Nursing Diagnoses

Potential for Infection transmission related to
contagious nature of organism
Altered Comfort: Headache, Fever, Neck Pain
related to meningeal irritation
Activity Intolerance related to fatigue and
malaise secondary to infection

Potential Impaired Skin Integrity related to
immobility, dehydration, and diaphoresis

Potential Altered Oral Mucous Membrane
related to dehydration and impaired ability
to perform mouth care

Potential Altered Nutrition: Less Than Body
Requirements related to anorexia, fatigue,
nausea, and vomiting

Potential Altered Respiratory Function related to
immobility and pain

Potential for Injury related to restlessness and
disorientation secondary to meningeal
irritation

Altered Family Processes related to critical
nature of situation and uncertain prognosis

Anxiety related to treatments, environment, and
risk of death

Potential Altered Health Maintenance related to
insufficient knowledge of: (specify)

Examples:

Condition	Signs and symptoms
Treatments	of complications
Pharmacologic	Follow-up care
therapy	Prevention of
Rest/activity	recurrence
balance	

SEXUALLY TRANSMITTED INFECTIOUS DISEASES (Venereal Diseases, Herpes)

Nursing Diagnoses

Potential for Infection Transmission related to
lack of knowledge of the contagious nature
of the disease

Fear related to nature of the condition and its
implications for life-style

Grieving related to chronicity of condition
(herpes)

Altered Comfort related to inflammatory process

Hopelessness related to incurable nature of
condition

Social Isolation related to fear of transmitting
disease to others

Potential Altered Health Maintenance related to
insufficient knowledge of: (specify)

Examples:
    Condition
    Modes of transmission
    Consequences of repeated infections
    Prevention of recurrences

ACQUIRED IMMUNODEFICIENCY SYNDROME (Adult)

See also End-Stage Cancer.

Collaborative Problems

Potential Complications:

Encephalopathy
Septicemia
Gastrointestinal bleeding
Pneumocystis carnii pneumonia
Meningitis
Esophagitis
Electrolyte imbalances

Nursing Diagnoses

Altered Comfort: Headache, Fever related to inflammation of cerebral tissue

Fatigue related to pulmonary insufficiency, chronic infections, malnutrition secondary to chronic diarrhea and gastrointestinal malabsorption

Potential Impaired Skin integrity related to perineal and anal tissue excoriation secondary to diarrhea and chronic genital candida or herpes lesions

Diarrhea related to unknown etiology

Altered Nutrition: Less Than Body Requirements related to chronic diarrhea, gastrointestinal malabsorption, fatigue, anorexia, and/or oral/esophageal lesions

Potential for Infection Transmission related to contagious nature of blood and body excretions

Social Isolation related to rejection of others after diagnosis

Hopelessness related to nature of the condition and poor prognosis

Potential Altered Health Maintenance related to
insufficient knowledge of: (specify)
Examples:
Condition
Medication therapy
Modes of transmission
Infection control
Community services

Neoplastic Disorders

CANCER (Initial Diagnosis)

See also specific types.

Nursing Diagnoses

Anxiety related to
Unfamiliar hospital environment
Uncertainty about cancer treatment outcomes
Feelings of loss and grief
Feelings of helplessness and/or hopelessness
Fear of death
Grieving of family members/significant others
related to
Changes in life-style or role relationship
Fear that patient will die
Powerlessness related to perceived loss or control
secondary to uncertainty about prognosis
and outcome of cancer treatment
Potential Altered Family Process related to
Examples:
Recent cancer diagnosis
Treatment plan creating significant changes
in life-style, role, or relationships
Little experience with losses
Nonsupportive family
High anxiety among family members and
patient
Immediate family includes children and
adolescents
Financial problems
Decisional Conflict related to treatment modality
choices

Potential Altered Health Maintenance related to
    insufficient knowledge of: (specify)
    Examples:
        Cancer
        Cancer treatment options
        Diagnostic tests
        Effects of treatment
        Treatment plan
        Support services related to
        Need for a new or different therapy

CANCER (General; Applies to Malignancies in Varied Sites and Stages)

Nursing Diagnoses

Altered Oral Mucous Membranes related to
    Examples:
        Disease process
        Therapy
            Radiation
            Chemotherapy
            Inadequate oral hygiene
            Altered nutritional/hydration status
    Potential Sexual Dysfunction related to (specify)
        or Potential Altered Sexuality Patterns
    Examples:
        Fear
        Grieving
        Changes in body image
        Anatomical changes
        Pain, fatigue (treatments, disease)
        Change in role responsibilities
Altered Comfort related to disease process and
    treatments
Diarrhea, related to
    Examples:
        Disease process   Radiation
        Chemotherapy   Medications
Colonic Constipation related to
    Examples:
        Disease process   Immobility
        Chemotherapy   Dietary intake
        Radiation therapy   Medications

Self-concept Disturbance related to
Examples:

Anatomical changes	Uncertain future
Role disturbances	Disruption of life-style

(Specify) Self-care Deficits related to fatigue,
pain, or depression

Potential for Infection related to altered immune
system

Altered Nutrition: Less Than Body
Requirements, related to anorexia, fatigue,
nausea, and vomiting secondary to disease
process and treatments

Potential for Injury: Physical Falls related to
Examples:
Disorientation
Weakness
Sensory–perceptual deterioration
Skeletal/muscle deterioration

Potential For Disuse Syndrome related to effects
of immobility

Altered nutrition status	Excretions/secretions
Altered circulation	Radiation therapy

Potential Fluid Volume Deficit related to
Examples:

Altered ability/desire to obtain fluids	Vomiting
	Diarrhea
	Depression
Weakness	Fatigue

Potential Impaired Home Maintenance
Management related to
Examples:
Lack of knowledge
Lack of resources
Support system
Equipment
Finances
Motor deficits
Sensory deficits
Cognitive deficits
Emotional deficits

Potential Impaired Social Interactions related to

fear of rejection or actual rejection of others
after diagnosis

Potential for Injury related to bleeding
tendencies and thrombocytopenia

Powerlessness related to inability to control
situation

Altered Family Process related to
Examples:

| Stress of diagnosis/ treatments | Role disturbances Uncertain future |

Grieving (Family, Individual) related to actual,
perceived, or anticipated losses associated
with diagnosis

Potential Altered Health Maintenance related to
insufficient knowledge of: (specify)
Examples:
Disease
Misconceptions
Treatments
Home care
Support agencies
Self-help groups
American Cancer Society
Hospital associations

CANCER (End-stage)

See also specific types.

Collaborative Problems

Potential Complications:

Hypercalcemia
Intracerebral metastasis
Malignant effusions
Narcotic toxicity
Pathological fractures
Spinal cord compression
Superior vena cava syndrome

Nursing Diagnoses

Altered Nutrition: Less Than Body
Requirements related to decreased oral
intake and increased metabolic rate

Colonic Constipation related to decreased
dietary fiber intake, decreased intestinal

mobility secondary to narcotic medication,
and inactivity

Pain related to inadequate relief from measures

Pruritus related to dry skin and biliary
obstruction

Ineffective Airway Clearance related to inability
to cough up secretions secondary to
weakness, increased viscosity, and pain

Impaired Physical Mobility related to pain,
sedation, weakness, fatigue, and edema

Potential for Injury related to weakness, fatigue,
and/or confusion

(Specify) Self-care Deficit related to fatigue,
weakness, sedation, pain, and/or decreased
sensory–perceptual capacity

Activity Intolerance related to hypoxia, fatigue,
malnutrition, and decreased mobility

Grieving related to terminal illness and
impending death, functional losses, changes
in self-concept, and withdrawal of others

Hopelessness related to functional losses and/or
impending death

Self-concept Disturbance related to dependence
on others to meet basic needs and decrease
in functional ability

Powerlessness related to change from curative
status to palliative status

Altered Family Processes related to change of
member to a terminal status and concern
over ability to manage home care

Spiritual Distress related to fear of death,
overwhelming grief, belief system conflicts,
and unresolved relationship conflicts

Potential Altered Health Maintenance related to
insufficient knowledge of: (specify)
Examples:
Pain management
Home care

COLORECTAL CANCER
(Additional Nursing Diagnoses)

See also Cancer (General).

Potential Sexual Dysfunction (Male) related to
inability to have or sustain an erection

secondary to surgical procedure on perineal structures

Potential Altered Health Maintenance related to insufficient knowledge of: (specify)

Examples:

Preoperative procedures

Postoperative procedures

Ostomy care

Appliances

Irrigations

Dietary management

Signs and symptoms of complications

Surgical Procedures

GENERAL SURGERY

Preoperative Period

Nursing Diagnoses

Fear related to surgical experience, loss of control, and the unpredictable outcome

Knowledge Deficit: (specify)

Examples:

Preoperative procedures

Surgical permit

Diagnostic studies

Foley catheter

Diet and fluid restrictions

Medications

Skin preparation

Waiting area for family

Postoperative procedure

Disposition (recovery room, intensive care unit)

Medications for pain

Coughing-turning-leg exercises

Tubes/drain placement

NPO/diet restrictions

Bed rest

Postoperative Period

Collaborative Problems

Potential Complications:

Urinary retention	*Peritonitis*
Hemorrhage	*Thrombophlebitis*
Hypovolemia/shock	*Paralytic ileus*
Renal failure	*Evisceration*
Pneumonia (stasis)	*Dehiscence*

Nursing Diagnoses

Potential for Infection related to destruction of first line of defense against bacterial invasion

Potential Altered Respiratory Function related to postanesthesia state, postoperative immobility, and pain

Acute Pain related to surgical interruption of body structures, flatus, and immobility

Impaired Physical Mobility related to pain and weakness secondary to anesthesia, tissue hypoxia, and insufficient fluids/nutrients

(Specify) Self-care Deficits related to limited mobility and pain

Potential Colonic Constipation related to decreased peristalsis secondary to the effects of anesthesia, immobility, and pain medication

Altered Nutrition: Less Than Body Requirements related to increased protein/vitamin requirements for wound healing and decreased intake secondary to pain, nausea, vomiting, and diet restrictions

Potential Altered Health Maintenance related to insufficient knowledge of: (specify)

Examples:

Home care	Activity
Incisional care	restriction
Signs and	Follow-up care
symptoms of	
complications	

AMPUTATION (Lower Extremity)

Preoperative Period

See Surgery (General).

Nursing Diagnoses

Anxiety related to lack of knowledge of:
Examples:
Postoperative routines
Postoperative sensations
Crutch-walking

Postoperative Period

Collaborative Problems

Potential Complications:

Edema of stump
Hemorrhage
Hematoma site

Nursing Diagnoses

Potential for Contractures related to impaired movement secondary to pain

Grieving related to loss of limb and its effects on life-style

Altered Comfort: Phantom Sensations related to nerve stimulation secondary to amputation

Potential for Injury related to altered gait and hazards of assistive devices

Potential Impaired Home Maintenance Management related to architectural barriers

Potential Altered Health Maintenance related to insufficient knowledge of: (specify)
Examples:
Adaptions in activities of daily living
Stump care
Prosthesis care
Gait training

ANEURYSM RESECTION (Abdominal Aortic)

See Surgery (General).

Preoperative Period
Collaborative Problems

Potential Complication: *Rupture of aneurysm*

Postoperative Period
Collaborative Problems

Potential Complications:

  Distal vessel thrombosis or emboli
  Renal failure
  Mesenteric ischemia/thrombosis
  Spinal cord ischemia

Nursing Diagnoses

Potential for Infection related to location of
    surgical incision
Potential Sexual Dysfunction (Male) related to
    possible loss of ejaculate and erections
    secondary to surgery and/or atherosclerosis
Potential Altered Health Maintenance related to
    insufficient knowledge of: (specify)
  Examples:
    Home care
    Activity restrictions
    Signs and symptoms of complications
    Follow-up care

ANORECTAL SURGERY

See also Surgery (General).

Preoperative Period (see Hemorrhoids
or Anal Fissure)

Postoperative Period
Collaborative Problems

Potential Complication: *Hemorrhage*
Potential Complication: *Urinary retention*

Nursing Diagnoses

Acute Pain related to surgical incision and
    spasms (sphincter, muscle)
Potential Constipation related to failure to
    respond to cues for defecation for fear of
    pain
Potential for Infection: Anal Area related to
    surgical incision and fecal contamination

Potential Altered Health Maintenance related to
insufficient knowledge of: (specify)
Examples:
Wound care
Prevention of recurrence
Nutritional requirements
Diet
Fluid
Exercise program
Signs and symptoms of complications

ARTERIAL BYPASS GRAFT OF LOWER EXTREMITY

(Aortic, Iliac, Femoral, Popliteal)

See also Surgery (General).
See also Anticoagulant Therapy.

Postoperative Period
Collaborative Problems

Potential Complications:

Thrombosis of graft
Compartmental syndrome
Lymphocele
Disruption of anastomosis

Nursing Diagnoses

Potential for Infection related to location of
surgical incision
Acute Pain related to increased tissue perfusion
to previously ischemic tissue
Potential Impaired Tissue Integrity related to
immobility and vulnerability of heels
Potential Altered Health Maintenance related to
insufficient knowledge of: (specify)
Examples:
Wound care
Signs and symptoms of complications
Activity restrictions
Follow-up care

ARTHROPLASTY (Total Hip, Knee, or Ankle Replacement)

Preoperative Period

See also Surgery (General).

Nursing Diagnoses

Anxiety related to lack of knowledge of use of trapeze

Postoperative Period

Collaborative Problems

Potential Complications:

Fat emboli
Hematoma formation
Infection
Dislocation of joint

Stress fractures
Neurovascular
  alterations
Synovial herniation
Thromboemboli
  formation

Nursing Diagnoses

Potential Impaired Skin Integrity related to immobility and incision

Activity Intolerance related to fatigue, pain, and impaired gait

Impaired Home Maintenance Management related to postoperative flexion restrictions

Potential Colonic Constipation related to activity restriction

Potential for Injury related to altered gait and assistive devices

Potential Altered Health Maintenance related to insufficient knowledge of: (specify)

Examples:
  Activity restrictions
  Use of supportive devices
    Walker
    Crutches
    Canes
  Rehabilitative program
  Follow-up care
  Apparel restrictions
  Signs of complications
  Supportive services
  Prevention of infection

ARTHROSCOPY, ARTHROTOMY, MENISCECTOMY, BUNIONECTOMY

See also Surgery (General).

Preoperative Period

Nursing Diagnoses

Anxiety related to lack of knowledge of crutch-walking and leg exercises

Postoperative Period

Collaborative Problems

Potential Complications:

Hematoma formation   Hemorrhage
Neurovascular   Effusion
   impairments

Nursing Diagnoses

Potential Altered Health Maintenance related to insufficient knowledge of: (specify)
   Examples:
      Home care
      Incision care
      Activity restrictions
      Signs of complications
      Follow-up care

CAROTID ENDARTERECTOMY

See also Surgery (General).

Postoperative Period

Collaborative Problems

Potential Complications:

Circulatory
   Thrombosis
   Hypotension
   Hypertension
   Hemorrhage
   Cerebral infarction
Neurological
   Cerebral infarction
   Cranial nerve impairment
      Facial
      Hypoglossal

Glosspharyngeal
Vagus
Local nerve impairment (peri-incisional
   numbness of skin)
Respiratory obstruction

Nursing Diagnoses

Potential for Injury related to syncope secondary
   to vascular insufficiency
Potential Altered Health Maintenance related to
   insufficient knowledge of: (specify)
   Examples:
      Risk factors
         Smoking
         Diet
         Obesity
      Activity restrictions
      Surgical site care
      Signs of complications
      Follow-up care

CATARACT EXTRACTION

Preoperative Period

Nursing Diagnoses

Fear related to upcoming surgery and potential
   failure to regain vision
Potential Altered Health Maintenance related to
   insufficient knowledge of: (specify)
   Examples:
      Preoperative routine
      Intra-operative experience
      Postoperative activities

Postoperative Period

Collaborative Problems

Potential Complication: Hemorrhage

Nursing Diagnoses

Acute Pain related to surgical interruption of
   body tissues
Potential for Infection related to increased

susceptibility secondary to surgical interruption of body surface

Potential for Injury related to visual limitations, unfamiliar environment, limited mobility, and postoperative eye patch

Potential Social Isolation related to altered visual acuity and fear of falling

Potential Impaired Home Maintenance Management related to inability to perform activities of daily living secondary to activity restrictions and visual limitations

Potential Altered Health Maintenance related to insufficient knowledge of: (specify)
> Examples:
>> Activities permitted and restricted
>> Medications
>> Complications (potential)
>> Follow-up care

CESAREAN SECTION

See also Surgery (General).
See Postpartum Period.

CESIUM IMPLANT

Preoperative Period

Nursing Diagnoses

Anxiety related to lack of knowledge of:
> Examples:
>> Internal radiation
>> Effects of internal radiation
>> Procedure
>> Precautions regarding caregivers/visitors
>> Activity restrictions

Postoperative Period

Collaborative Problems

Potential Complications:

> *Bleeding*
> *Infection*
> *Pulmonary complications*

Vaginal Stenosis
Radiation cystitis
Displacement of radioactive source
Thrombophlebitis
Bowel dysfunction

Nursing Diagnoses

Anxiety related to fear of radiation and its effects, uncertainty of outcome, feelings of isolation, and pain/or discomfort

Bathing, Toileting Self-care Deficit related to activity restrictions and isolation

Potential Impaired Skin Integrity related to immobility secondary to prescribed activity restrictions

Social Isolation related to precautions necessitated by cesium implant safety precautions

Potential Altered Health Maintenance related to insufficient knowledge of: (specify)
Examples:
Home care
Reportable signs and symptoms
Activity restrictions

CHOLECYSTECTOMY

See also Surgery (General).

Preoperative Period

Collaborative Problems

Potential Complication: Peritonitis

Nursing Diagnoses

Potential Altered Respiratory Function related to high abdominal incision and splinting secondary to pain

Potential Altered Oral Mucous Membrane related to NPO state and mouth breathing secondary to nasogastric intubation

COLOSTOMY

See also Surgery (General).

Preoperative Period

Nursing Diagnoses

Anxiety related to lack of knowledge of colostomy care and perceived negative effects on life-style

Postoperative Period

Collaborative Problems

Potential Complication: Peristomal ulceration/herniation
Potential Complication: Stomal necrosis, retraction, prolapse, stenosis, obstruction

Nursing Diagnoses

Grieving related to implications of cancer diagnosis

Potential Self-concept Disturbance related to effects of ostomy on body image

Potential Altered Sexuality Pattern related to perceived negative impact of ostomy on sexual functioning and attractiveness

Potential Sexual Dysfunction related to physiological impotence secondary to damaged sympathetic nerves (male) or inadequate vaginal lubrication

Potential Social Isolation related to anxiety over possible odor and leakage from appliance

Potential Altered Health Maintenance related to insufficient knowledge of: (specify)
Examples:
Stoma pouching procedure
Colostomy irrigation
Peristomal skin care
Perineal wound care
Incorporation of ostomy care into activities of daily living

CORNEAL TRANSPLANT (Penetrating Keratoplasty)

See also Surgery (General).

Preoperative Period

Nursing Diagnoses

Fear related to surgical experience, loss of
control, and unpredictable outcome
Anxiety related to lack of knowledge of:
Examples:
Preoperative routines
Postoperative routines/activities
Postoperative sensations

Postoperative Period

Collaborative Problems

Potential Complications:

Endophthalmitis
Increased intraocular pressure
Epithelial defects
Graft failure

Nursing Diagnoses

Potential for Infection related to nonintact
ocular defense mechanisms secondary to
surgery or previous eye disorder
Altered Comfort related to surgical procedure
Potential Altered Health Maintenance related to
insufficient knowledge of: (specify)
Examples:
Eye care
Resumption of activities
Medications/medication administration
Signs and symptoms of
Graft rejection
Glaucoma
Infection
Long term follow-up care

CORONARY ARTERY BYPASS GRAFT

See also Surgery (General).

Preprocedure Period

Nursing Diagnoses

Anxiety related to lack of knowledge of:
Pre–coronary artery bypass (CABG) routines/
care

CABG surgical procedure
Post-CABG routine/care
Fear (individual/family) related to the client's
health status, the need for CABG surgery,
and the unpredictable outcome

Postprocedure Period

Collaborative Problems

Potential Complications:

Cardiovascular insufficiency
Respiratory insufficiency
Renal insufficiency

Nursing Diagnoses

Acute Pain related to surgical incisions, chest
tubes, and immobility secondary to lengthy
surgery
Fear related to intensive environment of the
critical care unit and potential for
complications
Impaired Verbal Communication related to
endotracheal tube (temporary)
Altered Family Process related to disruption of
family life, fear of outcome (death,
disability), and stressful environment
(intensive care unit)
Potential Self-concept Disturbance related to the
symbolic meaning of the heart and changes
in life-style
Potential Altered Health Maintenance related to
insufficient knowledge of: (specify)
Examples:
Incisional care
Pain management (angina, incisions)
Signs and symptoms of complications
Condition
Pharmacologic care
Risk factors
Restrictions
Stress management techniques
Follow up care

CRANIAL SURGERY

See also Surgery (General).
See also Brain Tumor for preoperative/postoperative care.

Preoperative Period

Nursing Diagnoses

Anxiety related to impending surgery and
perceived negative effects on life-style

Postoperative Period

Collaborative Problems

Potential Complications:

Increased intracranial pressure
Cerebral edema
Hypoxia
Seizures
Brain hemorrhage, hematomas
Cranial nerve dysfunctions
Cardiac dysrhythmias
Fluid/electrolyte imbalances
Meningitis/encephalitis
Motor losses
Sensory losses
Speech losses
Memory losses
Cognitive losses
Perceptual losses
Hypothermia/hyperthermia
Antidiuretic hormone secretion disorders
Cerebrospinal fluid leaks
Hygromas
Brain shifts/herniations
Hydrocephalus
Gastrointestinal bleeding

Nursing Diagnoses

Altered Comfort: Headache related to
compression/displacement of brain tissue
and increased intracranial pressure
Potential Impaired Tissue Integrity: Corneal

related to inadequate lubrication secondary
to tissue edema

DILATATION AND CURETTAGE (D&C)

*See also Surgery (General; preoperative and
postoperative).*

Postoperative Period

Collaborative Problems

Potential Complication: Hemorrhage

Nursing Diagnoses

Potential Altered Health Maintenance related to
insufficient knowledge of: (specify)
Examples:
Condition
Home care

Signs and
symptoms of
complications
Activity
restrictions

ENUCLEATION

Preoperative Period

Nursing Diagnoses

Fear related to upcoming surgery, uncertain
outcome of surgery, and other factors
expressed by individual
Anxiety related to lack of knowledge of:
Preoperative routine
Intra-operative activities
Postoperative self-care activities

Postoperative Period

Collaborative Problems

Potential Complication: Hemorrhage

Nursing Diagnoses

Potential for Infection related to increased
susceptibility secondary to surgical

interruption of body surface and use of
prosthesis (ocular)

Potential for Injury related to visual limitations
and presence in unfamiliar environment

Acute Pain related to surgical interruption of
body surfaces

Grieving related to loss of eye and its effects on
life-style

Potential Self-concept Disturbance related to
effects of change in appearance on life-style

Potential Social Isolation related to changes in
body image and altered vision

Potential Impaired Home Maintenance
Management related to inability to perform
activities of daily living secondary to change
in visual abilities

Potential Altered Health Maintenance related to
insufficient knowledge of: (specify)
Examples:
Activities permitted
Self-care activities
Medications
Complications
Plans for follow-up care

FRACTURED HIP

See also Surgery (General).

Preoperative Period

Nursing Diagnoses

Acute Pain related to trauma and muscle
spasms

Anxiety related to lack of knowledge of use
of trapeze

Postoperative Period

Collaborative Problems

Potential Complications:

Hemorrhage/shock
Pulmonary embolism
Sepsis
Fat emboli

Compartmental syndrome
Peroneal nerve palsy
Displacement of hip joint
Venous stasis/thrombosis
Avascular necrosis of femoral head

Nursing Diagnoses

Acute Pain related to trauma and muscle spasms

(Specify) Self-care Deficit related to prescribed activity restriction

Potential Colonic Constipation related to immobility

Fear related to anticipated postoperative dependence

Potential Impaired Skin Integrity related to immobility and urinary incontinence secondary to inability to reach toilet quickly enough between urge to void and need to void

Potential Altered Health Maintenance related to insufficient knowledge of: (specify)

Examples:
Activity restrictions
Assistive devices
Home care
Follow-up care
Supportive services

HYSTERECTOMY (Vaginal, Abdominal)

See also Surgery (General).

Postoperative Period

Collaborative Problems

Potential Complications:

Vaginal bleeding (post–packing removal)
Urinary retention (post–catheter removal)

Fistula formation
Deep vein thrombosis
Trauma (ureter, bladder, rectum)

Nursing Diagnoses

Potential for Infection related to surgical intervention and presence of urinary catheter

Potential Self-concept Disturbance related to implications of loss of body part

Potential Altered Sexuality Patterns related to personal significance of loss of body part and implications of loss on life-style

Grieving related to loss of body part and childbearing ability

Potential Altered Health Maintenance related to insufficient knowledge of: (specify)

Examples:
Perineal/incisional care
Signs of complications
Activity restrictions
Sexual
Activities of daily living
Occupational
Loss of menses
Follow-up care (routine gynecological exams)

LAMINECTOMY

See also Surgery (General).

Preoperative Period

Nursing Diagnoses

Anxiety/Fear related to possibility of postoperative paralysis

Anxiety related to lack of knowledge of:

Examples:

Postoperative care	Monitoring
Positioning	Logrolling

Postoperative Period

Collaborative Problems

Potential Complications:

Neurosensory impairments
Bowel/bladder dysfunction

Cord edema
Skeletal misalignment
Cerebrospinal fluid leakage
Hematoma

Nursing Diagnoses

Potential for Injury related to vertigo secondary to postural hypotension

Acute Pain related to muscle spasms (back, thigh) secondary to irritation of nerves during surgery

Impaired Physical Mobility related to treatment restrictions

Potential Diversional Activity Deficit related to monotony of immobility

(Specify) Self-care Deficit related to activity restrictions

Potential Altered Health Maintenance related to insufficient knowledge of: (specify)

Examples:

| Activity restrictions | Exercises |
| Immobilization devices | |

MASTECTOMY

See also Cancer (General).
See also Surgery (General).

Preoperative Period

Nursing Diagnoses

Fear related to perceived effects of mastectomy (immediate [pain, edema], post-discharge [relationships, work]), and prognosis

Postoperative Period

Nursing Diagnoses

Potential Impaired Physical Mobility (shoulder, arm) related to lymphedema, nerve/muscle damage, and pain

Potential for Injury (affected arm) related to compromised lymph, motor, and sensory function

Potential Self-concept Disturbance related to perceived negative effects of loss of functioning

Grieving related to loss of breast and change in appearance

Potential Altered Health Maintenance related to insufficient knowledge of: (specify)
Examples:
Wound care
Exercises
Breast prosthesis
Signs and symptoms of complications
Hand/arm precautions
Community resources
Follow-up care

OPHTHALMIC SURGERY

See also Surgery (General).

Preoperative Period

Nursing Diagnoses

Anxiety related to lack of knowledge of:
Examples:
Postoperative positioning
Postoperative eye care/bandaging
Postoperative activity restrictions
Positioning
Bending
Stooping
Straining

Fear/Anxiety related to having surgery with a local anesthetic, possible loss of vision, and fear of pain during procedure

Potential for Injury related to impaired vision and unfamiliar environment

Postoperative Period
Collaborative Problems

Potential Complications:

Wound dehiscence/evisceration
Increased intraocular pressure
Retinal detachment

Dislocation of lens implant
Choroidal hemorrhage
Endophthalmitis
Hyphema
Hypopyon
Blindness

Nursing Diagnoses

Potential for Infection related to increased
susceptibility secondary to interruption of
body surfaces

Acute Pain related to surgical interruption of eye
structure

Potential for Injury related to: (specify)
Examples:
Visual limitations
Presence in unfamiliar environment
Presence of eye patches postoperatively

Potential Feeding, Hygiene Self-care Deficit
related to activity restrictions, visual
impairment, or presence of eye patch(es).

Potential sensory–perceptual alteration related to
insufficient input secondary to impaired
vision and/or presence of unilateral/bilateral
eye patches

Potential Altered Health Maintenance related to
insufficient knowledge of: (specify)
Examples:
Activities permitted and restricted
Medications
Complications (potential)
Plans for follow-up care

OTIC SURGERY (Stapedectomy,
Tympanoplasty, Myringotomy, Tympanic
Mastoidectomy)

See also Surgery (General).

Preoperative Period

Nursing Diagnoses

Anxiety/Fear related to possibility of greater loss
of hearing after surgery

Postoperative Period

Collaborative Problems

Potential Complications:

Hemorrhage	*Infection*
Facial paralysis	*Impaired hearing/*
	deafness

Nursing Diagnoses

Impaired Communication related to decreased
    hearing
Potential Social Isolation related to
    embarrassment of not being able to hear in
    a social setting
Potential for Injury related to vertigo
Potential Altered Health Maintenance related to
    insufficient knowledge of: (specify)
  Examples:
  Signs and symptoms of complications
    Facial nerve injury
    Vertigo
    Tinnitus
    Gait disturbances
    Ear discharge
  Ear care
  Contraindications
    Swimming
    Shampooing
    Air flights
    Showering
    Nose blowing
    Sneezing
    Coughing
    Straining
  Follow-up care

RADICAL NECK DISSECTION

(Laryngectomy)

Preoperative Period

See also Surgery (General).
See also Cancer (General).
See also Tracheostomy.

Nursing Diagnoses

Anxiety related to impending surgery and
   implications of condition on life-style
Anxiety related to lack of knowledge of: (specify)
   Examples:
      Postoperative disposition (intensive care
         unit)
      Ability to communicate
         Reading
         Writing
      Tracheostomy

Postoperative Period

Collaborative Problems

Potential Complications:

Hypoxia	Carotid artery rupture
Flap rejection	Cranial nerve injury
Hemorrhage	Infection

Nursing Diagnoses

Potential Impaired Physical Mobility: Shoulder,
   Head related to removal of muscles, nerves,
   flap graft reconstruction, trauma secondary
   to surgery
Potential Self-concept Disturbance related to
   change in appearance
Potential Altered Health Maintenance related to
   insufficient knowledge of: (specify)
   Examples:
      Condition
      Home care
         Oral hygiene
         Suctioning techniques
         Tracheostomy care
         Humidification
      Contraindications (lifting)
      Signs and symptoms of complications
         Swelling
         Pain
         Difficulty swallowing
         Purulent sputum

Follow-up care
Identification card/medallion
Esophageal breathing
Community services (American Cancer
Society)

RADICAL VULVECTOMY

See also Surgery (General).
See also Anticoagulant Therapy.

Preoperative Period

Nursing Diagnoses

Anxiety related to lack of knowledge of
preoperative/postoperative routines and
perceived negative effects on life-style

Postoperative Period

Collaborative Problems

Potential Complications:

Hemorrhage/shock
Urinary retention
Sepsis
Pulmonary embolism
Thrombophlebitis

Nursing Diagnoses

Acute Pain related to effects of surgery
Grieving related to loss of body function and its
effects on life-style
Potential Altered Sexuality Patterns related to
perceived negative impact of surgery on
sexual functioning and attractiveness
Potential Altered Health Maintenance related to
insufficient knowledge of: (specify)
Examples:
Home care
Wound care
Self-catheterization

RENAL SURGERY (General, Percutaneous Nephrostomy/Extracorporeal Renal Surgery, Nephrectomy)

See also Surgery (General).

Collaborative Problems

Potential Complications:

> Hemorrhage
> Shock
> Paralytic ileus
> Pneumothorax
> Of nephrostomy tube (calculi, fistulae, kinks)

Nursing Diagnoses

> Acute Pain related to distention of renal capsule and incision
> Potential Altered Respiratory Function related to pain on breathing and coughing secondary to location of incision
> Potential Altered Health Maintenance related to insufficient knowledge of: (specify)
> > Examples:
> > > Nephrostomy care
> > > Signs and symptoms of complications

RENAL TRANSPLANT

See also Corticosteroid Therapy.
See also Surgery (General).

Collaborative Problems

Potential Complications:

> Hemodynamic instability
> Hypervolemia/hypovolemia
> Hypertension/hypotension
> Renal failure (donor kidney)
> > Examples:
> > > Ischemic damage prior to implantation
> > > Hematoma
> > > Rupture of anastomosis
> > > Bleeding at anastomosis
> > > Renal vein thrombosis

Renal artery stenosis
Blockage of ureter (kinks, clots)
Kinking of ureter, renal artery
Rejection of donor tissue
Excessive immunosuppression
Electrolyte imbalances (potassium, phosphate)
Deep vein thrombosis
Sepsis

Nursing Diagnoses

Potential for Infection related to altered immune system secondary to medications

Potential Altered Oral Mucous Membrane related to increased susceptibility to infection secondary to immunosuppression

Potential Self-concept Disturbance related to transplant experience and potential for rejection

Fear related to possibility of rejection and dying

Potential Noncompliance related to complexity of treatment regimen (diet, medications, record-keeping, weight, blood pressure, urine testing) and euphoria (post-transplant)

Potential Altered Health Maintenance related to insufficient knowledge of: (specify)

Examples:

Prevention of infection
Personal hygiene
Wound care
Avoidance of contagious agents
Activity progression
Dietary management
Daily recording
Intake
Output
Weights
Urine testing
Blood pressure
Temperature
Pharmacologic therapy
Purpose
Timing
Dosage

Precautionary measures
Potential adverse effects
Daily urine testing (protein)
Signs/symptoms of rejection/infection
Avoidance of pregnancy
Follow-up care
Community resources

THORACIC SURGERY

See also Surgery (General).
See also Mechanical Ventilation.

Preoperative Period

Nursing Diagnoses

Anxiety/Fear related to possible respiratory
difficulty after surgery
Anxiety related to lack of knowledge of: (specify)
Examples:
Drainage devices
Mechanical ventilation

Postoperative Period

Collaborative Problems

Potential Complications:

Atelectasis
Pneumonia
*Respiratory
insufficiency*
*Complications of chest
drainage*

Pneumothorax
Hemorrhage
Pulmonary embolus
*Subcutaneous
emphysema*
Mediastinal shift

Nursing Diagnoses

Ineffective Airway Clearance related to difficulty in
coughing secondary to pain
Acute Pain related to surgical intervention and
drainage tube(s)
Activity Intolerance related to reduction in exercise
capacity secondary to loss of alveolar
ventilation
Impaired Physical Mobility: Arm/Shoulder related

to muscle trauma secondary to surgery and
position restrictions
Potential Altered Health Maintenance related to
insufficient knowledge of: (specify)
Examples:
Condition
Pain management
Shoulder/arm exercises
Incisional care
Breathing exercises
Splinting
Environmental hazards
Dust
Smoke
Irritating chemicals
Crowds during epidemics of upper
respiratory infection
Prevention of infection
Nutritional needs
Rest versus activity
Respiratory toilet
Follow-up care

TONSILLECTOMY

See also Surgery (General).

Collaborative Problems

Potential Complications:

Airway obstruction   Aspiration
Hemorrhage

Nursing Diagnoses

Potential Fluid Volume Deficit related to
decreased fluid intake secondary to pain on
swallowing
Potential Altered Nutrition: Less Than Body
Requirements related to decreased intake
secondary to pain on swallowing
Potential Altered Health Maintenance related to
insufficient knowledge of: (specify)
Examples:
Rest requirements

Nutritional needs
  Soft foods
  Fluids
Signs and symptoms of complications
    (hemorrhage)
Pain management
Positioning
Activity restrictions

TRANSURETHRAL RESECTION

(Prostate [Benign Hypertrophy or Cancer], Bladder Tumor)

See also Surgery (General).

Preoperative Period

Nursing Diagnoses

Anxiety related to lack of knowledge of: (specify)
  Examples:
    Postoperative procedures
      Foley catheter
      Genitourinary irrigation
      Nephrostomy/pyelostomy tubes
    Activity restrictions
    Oral fluid requirements

Postoperative Period

Collaborative Problems

Potential Complications:

Oliguria/anuria	Hyponatremia
Hemorrhage	Sepsis
Perforated bladder	Occlusion of drainage
(intraoperative)	devices

Nursing Diagnoses

Acute Pain and back/leg pains related to bladder
    spasms or clot retention
Potential Altered Sexuality Patterns related to
    fear of impotence resulting from surgical
    intervention
Potential Altered Health Maintenance related to
    insufficient knowledge of: (specify)

Examples:
Fluid requirements
Activity restrictions
Catheter care
Urinary control
Follow-up care

UROSTOMY

See also Surgery (General).

Preoperative Period

Nursing Diagnoses

Anxiety related to lack of knowledge of
urostomy care and perceived negative
effects on life-style

Postoperative Period

Collaborative Problems

Potential Complications:

Internal urine leakage
Urinary tract infection
Peristomal ulceration/herniation
Stomal necrosis, retraction, prolapse, stenosis,
obstruction

Nursing Diagnoses

Potential Self-concept Disturbance related to
effects of ostomy on body image
Potential Altered Sexuality Patterns related to
perceived negative impact of ostomy on
sexual functioning and attractiveness
Potential Sexual Dysfunction related to erectile
dysfunction (male) or inadequate vaginal
lubrication (female)
Potential Social Isolation related to anxiety over
possible odor and leakage from appliance
Potential Altered Health Maintenance related to
insufficient knowledge of: (specify)
Examples:
Stoma pouching procedure
Colostomy irrigation

Peristomal skin care
Perineal wound care
Incorporation of ostomy care into activities of daily living
Intermittent self-catheterization of Kock continent urostomy

Obstetrical/ Gynecological Conditions

Obstetrical Conditions

PRENATAL PERIOD (General)

Nursing Diagnoses

Nausea/Vomiting related to elevated estrogen levels, decreased blood sugar, or decreased gastric motility

Altered Comfort: Heartburn related to pressure on cardiac sphincter from enlarged uterus

Colonic Constipation related to decreased gastric motility and pressure of uterus on lower colon

Activity Intolerance related to fatigue and dyspnea secondary to pressure of enlarging uterus on diaphragm and increased blood volume

Potential Altered Oral Mucous Membranes related to hyperemic gums secondary to estrogen and progesterone levels

Fear related to the possibility of having an imperfect baby

Potential for Infection: Vaginal related to increased vaginal secretions secondary to hormonal changes

Potential for Injury related to syncope/

hypotension secondary to peripheral venous pooling

Altered Comfort: Headaches related to increased blood volume

Altered Comfort: Hemorrhoids related to constipation and increased pressure of enlarging uterus

Potential Self-concept Disturbance related to effects of pregnancy on biopsychosocial patterns

Potential Altered Parenting (mother, father) related to

Examples:

Knowledge deficit	Powerlessness
Unwanted pregnancy	Feelings of incompetence

Potential Altered Health Maintenance related to insufficient knowledge of: (specify)

Examples:

Effects of pregnancy on
  Body systems
    Cardiovascular
    Integumentary
    Gastrointestinal
    Urinary
    Pulmonary
    Musculoskeletal
  Psychosocial domain
  Sexuality/sexual function
  Family unit
    Spouse
    Children
Fetal growth and development
Nutritional requirements
Hazards of
  Smoking
  Excessive alcohol intake
  Drug abuse
  Excessive caffeine intake
  Excessive weight gain
Signs and symptoms of complications:
  Vaginal bleeding
  Cramping
  Gestational diabetes

Excessive edema
Preeclampsia
Preparation for childbirth
Classes
Printed references

ABORTION, INDUCED

Preprocedure Period

Nursing Diagnoses

Anxiety related to lack of knowledge of: (specify)
Examples:
Options available
Procedure
Postprocedure care
Normalcy of emotions

Postprocedure Period

Potential Ineffective Individual Coping related to
unresolved emotional responses (guilt) to
societal, moral, religious, and familial
opposition

Potential Altered Family Processes related to
effects of procedure on relationships
(disagreement regarding decisions, previous
conflicts [personal, marital], or adolescent
identity problems)

Potential Altered Health Maintenance related to
insufficient knowledge of: (specify)
Examples:
Self-care
Hygiene
Breast care
Nutritional needs
Expected bleeding, cramping
Signs and symptoms of complications
Resumption of sexual activity
Contraception
Sex education as indicated
Comfort measures
Expected emotional responses
Follow-up appointment
Community resources

ABORTION, SPONTANEOUS

Nursing Diagnoses

Fear related to possibility of subsequent
    abortions
Grieving related to loss of pregnancy

EXTRAUTERINE PREGNANCY

(Ectopic Pregnancy)

Collaborative Problems

Potential Complications:

Hemorrhage   *Sepsis*
Shock

Nursing Diagnoses

Grieving related to loss of fetus
Fear related to possibility of not being able to
    carry subsequent pregnancies
Acute Pain related to rupture of fallopian tube

HYPEREMESIS GRAVIDARUM

Collaborative Problems

Potential Complication: *Dehydration*
Potential Complication: *Negative nitrogen balance*

Nursing Diagnoses

Potential Altered Nutrition: Less Than Body
    Requirements related to loss of nutrients
    and fluid secondary to vomiting
Anxiety related to ambivalent feeling toward
    pregnancy and parenthood

TOXEMIA

See also Prenatal Period.
See also Postpartum Period.

Collaborative Problems

Potential Complications:

Hypertension   *Proteinuria*
Seizures   *Visual disturbances*

| Coma | Cerebral edema |
| Renal failure | Fetal compromise |

Nursing Diagnoses

Activity Intolerance related to compromised oxygen supply

Fear related to the effects of condition on self, pregnancy, and infant

Potential Impaired Skin Integrity related to generalized edema

Fluid Volume Excess: Edema related to retention of water and impairment of sodium excretion secondary to impaired renal function

Potential for Injury related to vertigo, visual disturbances, or seizures

Potential Altered Health Maintenance related to insufficient knowledge of: (specify)

Examples:

Dietary restrictions	Pharmacologic therapy
Signs and symptoms of complications	Comfort measures (headaches, backaches)
Conservation of energy	

UTERINE BLEEDING DURING PREGNANCY (Placenta Previa, Abruptio Placentae, Uterine Rupture, Nonmalignant Lesions, Hydatidiform Mole)

See also Postpartum Period.

Collaborative Problems

Potential Complications:

Hemorrhage	Renal failure
Shock	Fetal death
Disseminated intravascular coagulation	Anemia
	Sepsis

Nursing Diagnoses

Fear related to effects of bleeding on pregnancy and infant

Activity Intolerance related to the increased bleeding in response to activity

Grieving related to anticipated loss of pregnancy and loss of expected child

Fear related to possibility of subsequent future complications of pregnancy

INTRAPARTUM PERIOD (General)

Collaborative Problems

Potential Complications:

Hemorrhage (placenta previa, abruptio placentae)

Fetal distress
Hypertension
Uterine rupture

Nursing Diagnoses

Altered Comfort related to uterine contractions during labor

Fear related to unpredictability of uterine contractions and possibility of having an impaired baby

Potential Altered Health Maintenance related to insufficient knowledge of: (specify)
Examples:
Relaxation/breathing exercises
Positioning
Procedures
Preparations (bowel, skin)
Frequent assessments
Anesthesia (regional, inhalation)

POSTPARTUM PERIOD (General, Mastitis [Lactational], Fetal/Newborn Death)

General Postpartum Period

Collaborative Problems

Potential Complications:

Hemorrhage
Uterine atony

Retained placental fragments

Lacerations   Urinary retention
Hematomas

Nursing Diagnoses

Potential for Infection: Vaginal, Perineal related
 to bacterial invasion secondary to trauma
 during labor, delivery, and episiotomy
Potential for Infection: Breast related to milk
 production and trauma during breastfeeding
Potential Ineffective Breastfeeding related to
 Examples:
  Inexperience
  Engorged breasts
Altered Comfort related to
 Examples:

Trauma to	Hemorrhoids
perineum	Engorged breasts
during labor	Involution of
and delivery	uterus

Potential Colonic Constipation related to
 decreased intestinal peristalsis (postdelivery)
 and decreased activity
Potential Altered Parenting related to
 Examples:

Inexperience	Unwanted child
Feelings of	Disappointment
incompetence	with child
Powerlessness	Lack of role
	models

Stress Incontinence related to tissue trauma
 during delivery
Potential Sleep Pattern Disturbance related to
 maternity department's routines and
 demands of newborn
Situational Low Self-esteem related to changes
 that persist after delivery (skin, weight, and
 life-style)
Potential Altered Health Maintenance related to
 insufficient knowledge of: (specify)
 Examples:
  Postpartum routines
  Hygiene
   Breast
   Perineum

Exercises
Sexual counseling (contraception)
Nutritional requirements (infant, maternal)
Infant care
Stresses of parenthood
Adaptation of fathers
Sibling relationships
Parent/infant bonding
Postpartum emotional responses
Sleep/rest requirements
Household management
Community resources
Management of discomforts
  Breast
  Perineum
Social requirements
  Mother
  Couple
Signs and symptoms of complications

Mastitis (Lactational)

Collaborative Problems

Potential Complication: Abscess

Nursing Diagnoses

Acute Pain related to inflammation of breast
    tissue
Potential Ineffective Breastfeeding related to
    interruption secondary to inflammation
Potential Altered Health Maintenance related to
    insufficient knowledge of: (specify)
  Examples:
  Need for breast support
  Breast hygiene
  Breastfeeding restrictions
  Signs and symptoms of abscess formation

Fetal/Newborn Death

Nursing Diagnoses

Altered Family Processes related to emotional
    trauma of loss on each family member
Grieving related to loss of child

Fear related to the possibility of future fetal
deaths

CONCOMITANT MEDICAL CONDITIONS
(Cardiac Disease [Prenatal, Postpartum],
Diabetes [Prenatal, Postpartum])

Cardiac Disease

See also Cardiac Disorders.
See also Prenatal Period.
See also Postpartum Period.

Collaborative Problems

Potential Complications:

Congestive heart   Eclampsia
   failure   Valvular damage
Toxemia

Nursing Diagnoses

Fear related to effects of condition on self,
     pregnancy, and infant
Activity Intolerance related to increased
     metabolic requirements (pregnancy) in
     presence of compromised cardiac function
Impaired Home Maintenance Management
     related to impaired ability to perform role
     responsibilities during and after pregnancy
Potential Altered Family Processes related to
     disruption of activity restrictions and fears
     of effects on life-style
Potential Altered Health Maintenance related to
     insufficient knowledge of: (specify)
  Examples:
  Dietary   Signs and
     requirements   symptoms of
     (iron,   complications
     protein)   Community
  Prevention of   resources
     infection
  Conservation of
     energy

Diabetes (Prenatal)

See also Prenatal Period.
See also Diabetes Mellitus.
See also Postpartum Period.

Collaborative Problems

Potential Complications:

Hypoglycemia/   Acidosis
   hyperglycemia   Toxemia
Hydramnios

Nursing Diagnoses

Potential Impaired Skin Integrity related to
   excessive skin stretching secondary to
   hydramnios
Potential for Infection: Vaginal related to
   susceptibility to monilial infection
Altered Comfort: Headaches related to cerebral
   edema or hyperirritability
Potential Altered Health Maintenance related to
   insufficient knowledge of: (specify)
   Examples:
      Effects of pregnancy on diabetes
      Effects of diabetes on pregnancy
      Nutritional requirements
      Insulin requirements
      Signs and symptoms of complications
      Frequent blood/urine samples

Diabetes (Postpartum)

See also Postpartum Period (General).

Collaborative Problems

Potential Complications:

Hypoglycemia   Hemorrhage
Hyperglycemia   (secondary to
Toxemia   uterine atony from
Eclampsia   excessive amniotic
                         fluid)

Nursing Diagnoses

Anxiety related to separation from infant
   secondary to the need for special care needs
   of infant
Potential for Infection: Perineal Area related to
   depleted host defenses and depressed
   leukocytic phagocytosis secondary to
   hyperglycemia
Potential Altered Health Maintenance related to
   insufficient knowledge of: (specify)
   Examples:
      Risks of future pregnancies
      Birth control methods
         types contraindicated
      Special care requirements for infant

Gynecological Conditions

ENDOMETRIOSIS

Collaborative Problems

Potential Complication: Hypermenorrhea
Potential Complication: Polymenorrhea

Nursing Diagnoses

Chronic Pain related to response of displaced
   endometrial tissue (abdominal, peritoneal)
   to cyclic ovarian hormonal stimulation
Sexual Dysfunction related to painful intercourse
   or infertility
Anxiety related to unpredictable nature of
   disease
Potential Altered Health Maintenance related to
   insufficient knowledge of: (specify)
   Examples:
      Condition   Potential for
      Myths   pregnancy
      Pharmacologic
         therapy

REPRODUCTIVE TRACT INFECTIONS

(Vaginitis, Endometritis, Pelvic
Cellulitis, Peritonitis)

Collaborative Problems

Potential Complications:

Septicemia	Pneumonia
Abscess formation	Pulmonary embolism

Nursing Diagnoses

Altered Comfort related to infectious process

Potential Fluid Volume Deficit related to
inadequate intake, fatigue, pain, and fluid
losses secondary to elevated temperature

Potential Ineffective Individual Coping:
Depression related to chronicity of
condition and lack of definitive diagnosis/
treatment

Potential Altered Body Temperature related to
infectious process

Potential Altered Health Maintenance related to
insufficient knowledge of: (specify)

Examples:

Condition	Signs and
Nutritional	symptoms of
requirements	recurrence/
	complications
	Sleep/rest
	requirements

Neonatal Conditions

NEONATE, NORMAL

Collaborative Problems

Potential Complications:

Hypothermia
Hypoglycemia

Hyperbilirubinemia
Bradycardia

Nursing Diagnoses

Potential for Infection (Nosocomial) related to
　Vulnerability of infant
　Lack of normal flora
　Environmental hazards
　　Personnel　　　　　　Open wounds
　　Other newborns　　　　Umbilical cord
　　Parents　　　　　　　Circumcision
Potential Ineffective Airway Clearance related to
　oropharynx secretions
Potential Impaired Skin Integrity related to
　susceptibility to nosocomial infection and
　lack of normal skin flora
Ineffective Thermoregulation related to newborn
　extrauterine transition
Potential Altered Health Maintenance related to
　insufficient knowledge of: (specify) (see
　Postpartum Period)

NEONATE, PREMATURE

See also Family of High-risk Neonate.

Collaborative Problems

Potential Complications:

Cold stress　　　　　Hypocalcemia
Apnea　　　　　　　Sepsis
Bradycardia　　　　　Seizures
Hypoglycemia　　　　Pneumonia
Acidosis　　　　　　Hyperbilirubinemia

Nursing Diagnoses

Potential Altered Nutrition: Less Than Body
　Requirements related to diminished sucking
Potential Colonic Constipation related to
　decreased intestinal motility and immobility
Potential for Aspiration related to immobility
　and increased secretions

Potential for Infection (Nosocomial) related to
    Vulnerability of infant
    Lack of normal flora
    Environmental hazards
    Personnel
    Other newborns
    Parents
    Open wounds
        Umbilical cord
        Circumcision
Potential Impaired Skin Integrity related to
    susceptibility to nosocomial infection (lack
    of normal skin flora)
Ineffective Thermoregulation related to newborn
    transition to extrauterine environment

NEONATE, POSTMATURE
(Small for Gestational Age [SGA],
Large for Gestational Age [LGA])

Collaborative Problems

Potential Complications:

Asphyxia at birth
Meconium aspiration
Hypoglycemia
Polycythemia (SGA)
Edema
   Generalized
   Cerebral
Central nervous system depression
Renal tubular necrosis
Impaired intestinal absorption
Birth injuries (LGA)

Nursing Diagnoses

Potential Impaired Skin Integrity related to
    absence of protective vernix and prolonged
    exposure to amniotic fluid (LGA)
Potential Altered Nutrition: Less Than Body
    Requirements related to swallowing and
    sucking difficulties

NEONATE WITH SPECIAL PROBLEM
(Congenital Infections—Cytomegalovirus
[CMV], Rubella, Toxoplasmosis,
Syphilis, Herpes)

See also High-risk Neonate.
See also Family of High-risk Neonate.
See also Developmental Problems/Needs under
  Pediatric Disorders.

Collaborative Problems

Potential Complications:

Hyperbilirubinemia	*Cataracts (rubella)*
Hepatosplenomegaly	*Retinitis*
Anemia	*Thrombocytopenic*
Hydrocephalus	*purpura (rubella)*
Microcephaly	*Sensory-motor*
Mental retardation	*deafness (CMV)*
Congenital heart	*Periostitis (syphilis)*
disease (rubella)	*Seizures*

Nursing Diagnoses

Potential for Infection Transmission related to
  contagious nature of organism
Potential for Injury related to uncontrolled tonic/
  clonic movements
Potential Altered Nutrition: Less Than Body
  Requirements related to poor sucking reflex

NEONATE OF A DIABETIC MOTHER

See also Neonate, Normal.
See also Family of High-risk Neonate.

Collaborative Problems

Potential Complications:

Hypoglycemia	*Acidosis*
Hypocalcemia	*Birth injury*
Polycythemia	*(macrosomia)*
Hyperbilirubinemia	*Hyaline membrane*
Sepsis	*disease (if*

| Respiratory distress | premature) |
| syndrome | Venous thrombosis |

Nursing Diagnoses

Potential Fluid Volume Deficit related to
increased urinary excretion and osmotic
diuresis

HIGH-RISK NEONATE

See also Family of High-risk Neonate.

Collaborative Problems

Potential Complications:

Hypoxia	Seizures
Shock	Hypotension
Respiratory distress	Septicemia

Nursing Diagnoses

Altered Comfort related to abdominal distention
Potential Altered Nutrition: Less Than Body
Requirements related to poor sucking reflex
secondary to (specify)
Potential for Injury related to uncontrolled
tonic/clonic movements or hyperirritability
Potential for Infection (Nosocomial) related to
Vulnerability of infant
Lack of normal flora
Environmental hazards
Personnel
Other newborns
Parents
Open wounds
Umbilical cord
Circumcision
Potential Altered Respiratory Function related to
oropharyngeal secretions
Potential Impaired Skin Integrity related to
susceptibility to nosocomial infection
secondary to lack of normal skin flora
Ineffective Thermoregulation related to newborn
transition to extrauterine environment

FAMILY OF HIGH-RISK NEONATE

Nursing Diagnoses

Grieving related to realization of present or future loss for family and/or child

Altered Family Processes related to effect of extended hospitalization on family (role responsibilities, finances)

Anxiety related to unpredictable prognosis

Potential Altered Parenting related to inadequate bonding secondary to parent–child separation or failure to accept impaired child

Ineffective Individual Coping related to perceived parental role failure

HYPERBILIRUBINEMIA (Rh Incompatibility, ABO Incompatibility)

See also Family of High-risk Neonate.
See also Neonate, Normal.

Collaborative Problems

Potential Complications:

Anemia
Jaundice
Kernicterus
Hepatosplenomegaly
Hydrops fetalis
(cardiac failure,
hypoxia, anasarca,
and pericardial,
pleural, and
peritoneal effusions)

Renal failure
(phototherapy
complications,
hyperthermia/
hypothermia,
dehydration,
priapism, "bronze
baby" syndrome)

Nursing Diagnoses

Potential Impaired Tissue Integrity: Corneal related to exposure to phototherapy light and continuous wearing of eye pads

Potential Impaired Skin Integrity related to diarrhea, urinary excretions of bilirubin, and exposure to phototherapy light

NEONATE OF NARCOTIC-ADDICTED MOTHER

See also Family of High-risk Neonate.
See also Neonate, Normal.
See also Substance Abuse for Mother.

Collaborative Problems

Potential Complications:

Hyperirritability/
    seizures
Withdrawal
Hypocalcemia
Hypoglycemia

Sepsis
Dehydration
Electrolyte imbalances
Aspiration

Nursing Diagnoses

Potential Altered Nutrition: Less Than Body
    Requirements related to uncoordinated and
    ineffective sucking and swallowing reflexes
Potential Impaired Skin Integrity related to
    generalized diaphoresis and marked rigidity
Diarrhea related to increased peristalsis
    secondary to hyperirritability
Sleep Pattern Disturbance related to
    hyperirritability
Potential for Injury: Blisters related to frantic
    sucking of fists
Potential for Injury related to uncontrolled
    tremors or tonic/clonic movements
Sensory–Perceptual Alterations related to
    hypersensitivity to environmental stimuli

RESPIRATORY DISTRESS SYNDROME

See also High-risk Neonate.
See also Mechanical Ventilation.

Collaborative Problems

Potential Complications:

Hypoxia
Atelectasis
Acidosis

Sepsis
Hyperthermia

Nursing Diagnoses

Activity Intolerance related to insufficient oxygenation of tissues secondary to impaired respirations

Potential for Infection (Nosocomial) related to vulnerability of infant, lack of normal flora, environmental hazards (personnel, other newborns, parents), and open wounds (umbilical cord, circumcision)

Potential Impaired Skin Integrity related to susceptibility to nosocomial infection and lack of normal skin flora

SEPSIS (Septicemia)

See also Newborn.
See also Family of High-risk Neonate.

Collaborative Problems

Potential Complications:

Anemia	Seizures
Respiratory distress	Hepatosplenomegaly
Hypothermia/	Hemorrhage
hyperthermia	Jaundice
Hypotension	Meningitis
Edema	Pyarthrosis

Nursing Diagnoses

Potential Impaired Skin Integrity related to edema and immobility

Altered Nutrition: Less Than Body Requirements related to poor sucking reflex

Diarrhea related to intestinal irritation secondary to infecting organism

Potential for Injury related to uncontrolled tonic/clonic movements

Potential for Injury: Ecchymosis related to hematopoietic insufficiency

Potential Altered Body Temperature related to body response to pathogens

Pediatric/Adolescent Disorders*

DEVELOPMENTAL PROBLEMS/NEEDS RELATED TO CHRONIC ILLNESS
(*e.g.,* Permanent Disability, Multiple Handicaps, Developmental Disability [Mental/Physical], Life-threatening Illness)

Nursing Diagnoses

Grieving (Parental) related to anticipated losses secondary to condition

Altered Family Processes related to adjustment requirements for situation

Examples:
Time
Energy
Emotional
Physical
Financial
Physical care

Potential Impaired Home Maintenance Management related to inadequate resources, housing, or impaired caregiver(s)

Potential Parental Role Conflict related to separations secondary to frequent hospitalizations

Potential Social Isolation (Child/Family) related to the disability and the requirements of the caregiver(s)

---

* For additional pediatric medical diagnoses, see the adult diagnoses and also Developmental Problems/Needs; for example:

Diabetes mellitus	Neoplastic disorders
Anorexia nervosa (psychiatric disorders)	Fractures
Spinal cord injury	Congestive heart failure
Head trauma	Pneumonia

Potential Altered Parenting related to abuse,
rejection, overprotection secondary to
inadequate resources or coping mechanisms

Decisional Conflict related to illness, health-care
interventions, and parent–child separation

(Specify) Self-care Deficit related to illness
limitations or hospitalization

Potential Altered Growth and Development
related to impaired ability to achieve
developmental tasks secondary to
restrictions imposed by disease, disability, or
treatments

ACQUIRED IMMUNODEFICIENCY
SYNDROME (Child)

*See also Acquired Immunodeficiency Syndrome
(Adult).*
*See also Development Problems/Needs Related to
Chronic Illness*

Nursing Diagnoses

Potential for Infection transmission related to
exposure to stool and other secretions
during diaper changes or failure of child to
follow handwashing procedure after
toileting

Altered Nutrition: Less Than Body
Requirements related to lactose intolerance,
need for double the usual recommended
daily allowance, anorexia secondary to oral
lesions, and malaise

Altered Growth and Development related to
decreased muscle tone secondary to
encephalopathy

Impaired Physical Mobility related to hypotonia
or hypertonia secondary to cortical atrophy

Altered Family Processes related to the impact of
the child's condition on role responsibilities,
siblings, finances, and negative responses of
relatives, friends, and community

Potential Altered Health Maintenance related to
insufficient knowledge of: (specify)

Examples:
  Modes of transmission
  Risks of live virus vaccines
  Avoidance of infections
  School attendance
  Community resources

ASTHMA

See also Developmental Problems/Needs.

Collaborative Problems

Potential Complications:

Hypoxia   *Respiratory acidosis*
Corticosteroid therapy

Nursing Diagnoses

Ineffective Airway Clearance related to
    bronchospasm and increased pulmonary
    secretions
Fear related to breathlessness and recurrences
Potential Altered Health Maintenance related to
    insufficient knowledge of: (specify)
  Examples:
    Condition
    Environmental hazards
      Smoking
      Allergens
      Weather
    Prevention of infection
    Breathing/relaxation exercises
    Signs and symptoms of complications
    Pharmacologic therapy
    Fluid requirements
    Behavioral modification
    Daily diary recording

CELIAC DISEASE

See also Developmental Problems/Needs.

Collaborative Problems

Potential Complications:

Severe malnutrition/ dehydration	Osteoporosis
Anemia	Electrolyte imbalances
Altered blood coagulation	Metabolic acidosis
	Shock
	Delayed growth

Nursing Diagnoses

Potential Altered Nutrition: Less Than Body Requirements related to malabsorption, dietary restrictions, and anorexia

Diarrhea related to decreased absorption in small intestines secondary to damaged villi resulting from toxins from undigested gliadin

Potential Fluid Volume Deficit related to fluid loss in diarrhea

Potential Altered Health Maintenance related to insufficient knowledge of: (specify)
    Examples:
        Dietary management
           Restrictions
           Vitamin
           Protein
           Carbohydrate requirements

CEREBRAL PALSY*

See also Developmental Problems/Needs.

Collaborative Problems

Potential Complications:

Contractures	Respiratory infections
Seizures	

* Because disabilities associated with cerebral palsy can be varied, (hemiparesis, quadriparesis, diplegia, monoplegeia, triplegia, paraplegia), the nurse will have to specify the child's limitations clearly in the diagnostic statements.

Nursing Diagnoses

Potential for Injury related to inability to control movements

Potential Altered Nutrition: Less Than Body Requirements related to sucking difficulties (infant) and dysphagia

(Specify) Self-care Deficit related to sensory-motor impairments

Impaired Verbal Communication related to impaired ability to speak words related to facial muscle involvement

Potential Fluid Volume Deficit related to difficulty obtaining or swallowing liquids

Potential Diversional Activity Deficit related to effects of limitations on ability to participate in recreational activities

Potential Altered Health Maintenance related to insufficient knowledge of: (specify)

Examples:

Disease	Education
Pharmacologic regime	Community services
Activity program	Orthopedic appliances

CHILD ABUSE (Battered Child Syndrome, Child Neglect)

See also Fractures, Burns.
See also Failure to Thrive.

Collaborative Problems

Potential Complications:

Trauma (fractures, burns, lacerations)
Failure to thrive
Malnutrition

Drug or alcohol addiction (older child)
Venereal disease
Pregnancy in young adolescent

Nursing Diagnoses

Ineffective Family Coping: Disabled related to presence of factors that contribute to child abuse

Examples:
    Lack of or unavailability of extended family
    Economic conditions
        Inflation
        Unemployment
    Lack of role model as a child
    High-risk children
        Unwanted
        Of undesired gender or appearance
        Physically or mentally handicapped
        Hyperactive
        Terminally ill
    High-risk parents
        Single
        Adolescent
        Emotionally disturbed
        Alcoholic
        Drug-addicted
        Physically ill
Ineffective Individual Coping (Child Abuser)
    related to
    Examples:
        History of abuse by own parents and lack of
            warmth and affection from them
        Social isolation (few friends or outlets for
            tensions)
        Marked lack of self-esteem, with low
            tolerance for criticism
        Emotional immaturity and dependency
        Distrust of others
        Inability to admit need for help
        High expectations for/of child (perceiving
            child as a source of emotional
            gratification)
    Unrealistic desire for child to give pleasure
Ineffective Individual Coping (nonabusing
    parent) related to passive and compliant
    response to abuse
Fear related to possibility of placement in a
    shelter or foster home
Fear (parental) related to responses of others,
    possible loss of child, and criminal
    prosecution
Potential Altered Nutrition: Less Than Body

Requirements related to inadequate intake
secondary to lack of knowledge or neglect
Potential Altered Health Maintenance related to
insufficient knowledge of: (specify)
Examples:
Parenting skills
Discipline
Expectations
Constructive stress management
Signs and symptoms of abuse
High-risk groups
Parent(s)
Child
Child protection laws
Community services
Hotlines
Counselling

CLEFT LIP AND PALATE

See also Developmental Problems/Needs.
See also Surgery (General).

Preoperative Period

Nursing Diagnoses

Potential Altered Nutrition: Less Than Body
Requirements related to inability to suck
secondary to cleft lip

Postoperative Period

Collaborative Problems

Potential Complication: *Respiratory distress*
Potential Complication: *Failure to thrive (organic)*

Nursing Diagnoses

Impaired Physical Mobility related to restricted
activity secondary to use of restraints
Potential Impaired Verbal Communication
related to impaired muscle development,
insufficient palate function, faulty dentition,
or hearing loss

Potential for Aspiration related to impaired
sucking
Potential Altered Health Maintenance related to
insufficient knowledge of: (specify)
Examples:
Condition
Feeding and suctioning techniques
Surgical site care
Risks for otitis media (dental/oral problems)
Referral to speech therapist

COMMUNICABLE DISEASES

See also Developmental Problems/Needs.

Nursing Diagnoses

Altered Comfort related to fatigue, malaise, sore
throat, elevated temperature
Potential for Infection Transmission related to
contagious agents
Potential Fluid Volume Deficit related to
increased fluid loss secondary to elevated
temperature or insufficient oral intake
secondary to malaise
Potential Altered Nutrition: Less Than Body
Requirements related to anorexia and sore
throat or pain on chewing (mumps)
Altered Comfort: Photophobia related to
disorder
Pruritus related to lesions
Potential Ineffective Airway Clearance related to
increased mucus production (whooping
cough)
Potential Altered Health Maintenance related to
insufficient knowledge of: (specify)
Examples:
Condition   Immunizations
Transmission   Skin care
Prevention

CONGENITAL HEART DISEASE

*See also Developmental Problems/Needs related to
chronic illness.*

Collaborative Problems

Potential Complications:

Congestive heart failure
Pneumonia
Hypoxemia
Cerebral thrombosis
Digoxin toxicity

Nursing Diagnoses

Activity Intolerance related to insufficient
    oxygenation secondary to heart defects
Potential Altered Nutrition: Less Than Body
    Requirements related to inadequate
    sucking, fatigue, and dyspnea
Potential Altered Health Maintenance related to
    insufficient knowledge of: (specify)
  Examples:
    Condition
    Prevention of infection
    Signs and symptoms of complications
    Digoxin therapy
    Nutrition requirements
    Community services

CONVULSIVE DISORDERS

See also Developmental Problems/Needs.
See also Mental Disabilities, if indicated.

Collaborative Problems

Potential Complication: Respiratory arrest
Potential Complication: Hypoxia

Nursing Diagnoses

Potential for Injury related to uncontrolled
    movements of seizure activity
Anxiety related to embarrassment and fear of
    seizure episodes
Potential Ineffective Individual Coping:
    Aggression related to restrictions, parental
    overprotection, parental indulgence
Potential Altered Health Maintenance related to
    insufficient knowledge of: (specify)

Examples:
Condition/cause
Pharmacologic therapy
Treatment during seizures
Seizure precautions
Environmental hazards
Water
Driving
Heights

CRANIOCEREBRAL TRAUMA

Collaborative Problems

Potential Complications:

Increased intracranial pressure
Hemorrhage
Tentorial herniation
Cranial nerve dysfunction

Nursing Diagnoses

Altered Comfort: Headache related to
compression/displacement of cerebral tissue
Potential for Injury related to uncontrolled
tonic/clonic movements during seizure
episode and/or somnolence
Potential Altered Health Maintenance related to
insufficient knowledge of: (specify)
Examples:
Condition
Signs and symptoms of complications
Posttraumatic syndrome
Activity restrictions
Follow-up care

CYSTIC FIBROSIS

See also Developmental Problems/Needs.

Collaborative Problems

Potential Complication: Bronchopneumonia, atelectasis
Potential Complication: Paralytic ileus

Nursing Diagnoses

Ineffective Airway Clearance related to
mucopurulent secretions

Potential Altered Nutrition: Less Than Body
Requirements related to need for increased
calories and protein secondary to impaired
intestinal absorption, loss of fat, and fat-
soluable vitamins in stools

Constipation/Diarrhea related to excessive or
insufficient pancreatic enzyme replacement

Activity Intolerance related to dyspnea
secondary to mucopurulent secretions

Potential Altered Health Maintenance related to
insufficient knowledge of: (specify)
Examples:
Condition (genetic transmission)
Risk for infection
Pharmacological therapy
Side-effects
Ototoxicity
Renal toxicity
Equipment
Oxygen
Nebulization
Nutritional therapy
Salt replacement requirements
Breathing exercises
Postural drainage
Exercise program
Community resources (Cystic Fibrosis
Foundation)

DOWN SYNDROME

See also Developmental Problems/Needs.
See also Mental Disabilities, if indicated.

Nursing Diagnoses

Potential Altered Respiratory Function related to
decreased respiratory expansion secondary
to decreased muscle tone, inadequate mucus
drainage, and mouth-breathing

Potential Impaired Skin Integrity related to

rough, dry skin surface and flaccid
extremities

Potential Colonic Constipation related to
decreased gastric motility

Altered Nutrition: Less Than Body
Requirements (infant) related to sucking
difficulties secondary to large, protruding
tongue

Potential Altered Nutrition: Greater Than Body
Requirements related to increased caloric
consumption secondary to boredom in the
presence of limited physical activity

(Specify) Self-care Deficits related to physical
limitations

Potential Altered Health Maintenance related to
insufficient knowledge of: (specify)
Examples:
Condition   Community
Home care   services
Education

FAILURE TO THRIVE (Nonorganic)

See also Developmental Problems/Needs.

Collaborative Problems

Potential Complication: Metabolic dysfunction
Potential Complication: Dehydration

Nursing Diagnoses

Ineffective Individual Coping (caregiver) related
to failure to respond to child's needs
(emotional/physical) secondary to
caregiver's emotional problems

Altered Nutrition: Less Than Body
Requirements related to inadequate intake
secondary to the lack of emotional and
sensory stimulation or lack of knowledge of
caregiver

Sensory–Perceptual Alterations related to history
of insufficient sensory input from primary
caregiver

Sleep Pattern Disturbance related to anxiety and

apprehension secondary to parental deprivation

Altered Parenting related to

Examples:

Lack of knowledge of parenting skills	Lack of role model
	Relationship problems
Impaired caregiver	Unrealistic expectations for child
Impaired child	
Lack of support system	Unmet psychological needs

Impaired Home Maintenance Management related to difficulty of caregiver with maintaining a safe home environment

Potential Altered Health Maintenance related to insufficient knowledge of: (specify)

Examples:

Growth and development requirements	Risk for child abuse
	Parenting skills
Feeding guidelines	Community agencies

GLOMERULAR DISORDERS

(Glomerulonephritis: Acute, Chronic; Nephrotic Syndrome: Congenital, Secondary, Idiopathic)

See also Developmental Problems/Needs.
See also Corticosteroid Therapy.

Collaborative Problems

Potential Complications:

Anasarca (generalized edema)	*Malnutrition*
	Ascites
Hypertension	*Pleural effusion*
Azotemia	*Hypoalbuminemia*
Septicemia	

Nursing Diagnoses

Potential for Infection related to increased
  susceptibility during edematous phase and
  lowered resistance secondary to
  corticosteroid therapy

Potential Impaired Skin Integrity related to
  Examples:

Immobility	Frequent
Lowered resistance	application of collection
Edema	bags

Altered Nutrition: Less Than Body
  Requirements related to dietary restrictions,
  anorexia secondary to fatigue, malaise, and
  pressure on abdominal structures (edema)

Fatigue related to circulatory toxins, fluid and
  electrolytic imbalance

Diversional Activity Deficit related to
  hospitalization and impaired ability to
  perform usual activities

Potential Altered Health Maintenance related to
  insufficient knowledge of: (specify)
  Examples:
    Condition
    Etiology
    Course
    Treatments
    Signs and symptoms of complications
    Pharmacologic therapy
    Nutritional/fluid requirements
    Prevention of infection
    Home care
      Diet
      Urine testing
      Follow-up care
      Community services

HEMOPHILIA

See also Developmental Problems/Needs.

Collaborative Problems

Potential Complication: Hemorrhage

Nursing Diagnoses

Acute/Chronic Pain related to joint swelling and limitations secondary to hemarthrosis

Potential Impaired Physical Mobility related to joint swelling and limitations secondary to hemarthrosis

Potential Altered Oral Mucous Membranes related to trauma from coarse food and insufficient dental hygiene

Potential Altered Health Maintenance related to insufficient knowledge of: (specify)

Examples:

Condition	Environmental
Contraindications	hazards
(*e.g.,* aspirin)	Emergency
Genetic	treatment to
transmission	control
	bleeding

HYDROCEPHALUS

See also Developmental Problems/Needs related to chronic illness.

Collaborative Problems

Potential Complication: Increased intracranial –pressure

Potential Complication: Sepsis (post-shunt procedure)

Nursing Diagnoses

Potential Impaired Skin Integrity related to impaired ability to move head secondary to size

Potential for Injury related to inability to support large head and strain on neck

Potential Altered Nutrition: Less Than Body Requirements related to vomiting secondary to cerebral compression and irritability

Potential Altered Health Maintenance related to insufficient knowledge of: (specify)

Examples:
Condition
Home care

Signs and symptoms of infection, increased
intracranial pressure
Emergency treatment of shunt

INFECTIOUS MONONUCLEOSIS

(Adolescent)

Collaborative Problems

Potential Complication: Enlarged spleen
Potential Complication: Hepatic dysfunction

Nursing Diagnoses

Activity Intolerance related to fatigue secondary
to infectious process

Acute Pain related to sore throat and headaches

Altered Health Maintenance related to need for
nutritional counseling and sleep
requirements

Potential Altered Nutrition: Less Than Body
Requirements related to sore throat and
malaise

Grieving related to restrictions of disease and
treatments on life-style

Potential for Infection Transmission related to
contagious condition

Potential Altered Health Maintenance related to
insufficient knowledge of: (specify)

Examples:
Condition
Communicable nature
Diet therapy
Risks of alcohol ingestion (with hepatic
dysfunction)
Signs and symptoms of complications
Hepatic
Splenic
Neurologic
Hematologic
Activity restrictions

LEGG-CALVÉ-PERTHES DISEASE

See also Developmental Problems/Needs.

Collaborative Problems

Potential Complication: Permanent deformed
femoral head

Nursing Diagnoses

Pain related to joint dysfunction
Potential Impaired Skin Integrity related to
immobilization devices (casts, braces)
(Specify) Self-care Deficits related to pain and
immobilization devices
Potential Altered Health Maintenance related to
insufficient knowledge of: (specify)
Examples:
Disease
Weight-bearing restrictions
Application/maintenance of devices
Pain management at home

LEUKEMIA

See also Chemotherapy.
See also Radiation Therapy.
See also Cancer (General).
See also Developmental Problems/Needs.

Collaborative Problems

Potential Complications:

Hepatosplenomegaly
Increased intracranial edema
Metastasis (brain, lungs, kidneys, gastrointestinal
tract, spleen, liver)
Hypermetabolism
Hemorrhage
Dehydration
Myelosuppression

Nursing Diagnoses

Potential for Infection related to altered immune
system secondary to leukemic process and
side-effects of chemotherapeutic agents
Potential Social Isolation related to effects of

disease and treatments on appearance and
fear of embarrassment
Potential Altered Growth and Development
related to impaired ability to achieve
developmental tasks secondary to
limitations of disease and treatments

MENINGITIS (Bacterial)

See also Developmental Problems/Needs.

Collaborative Problems

Potential Complications:

Peripheral circulatory collapse
Disseminated intravascular coagulation
Increased intracranial pressure/hydrocephalus
Visual/auditory nerve palsies
Paresis (hemi-, quadri-)
Subdural effusions
Respiratory distress
Seizures
Fluid/electrolyte imbalances

Nursing Diagnoses

Potential for Injury related to seizure activity
secondary to infectious process
Altered Comfort related to nuchal rigidity,
muscle aches, and immobility
Sensory–Perceptual Alteration: Visual, Auditory
related to increased sensitivity to external
stimuli secondary to infectious process
Impaired Physical Mobility related to
intravenous infusion, nuchal rigidity, and
restraining devices
Potential Impaired Skin Integrity related to
immobility
Potential Altered Body Temperature related to
infectious processes
Potential Altered Health Maintenance related to
insufficient knowledge of: (specify)
Examples:
Condition   Diagnostic
Antibiotic therapy   procedures

MENINGOMYELOCELE

See also Developmental Problems/Needs.

Collaborative Problems

Potential Complications:

Hydrocephalus/shunt infections
Increased intracranial pressure
Urinary tract infections

Nursing Diagnoses

Reflex Incontinence related to sensory-motor
dysfunction
Potential for Infection related to vulnerability of
meningomyelocele sac
Potential Impaired Skin Integrity related to
sensory-motor impairments and orthopedic
appliances
(Specify) Self-care Deficit related to sensory-
motor impairments
Potential for Injury: Fractures, Membrane Tears,
related to pathological condition
Impaired Physical Mobility related to lower limb
impairments
Grieving (parental) related to birth of infant with
defects
Potential Altered Health Maintenance related to
insufficient knowledge of: (specify)
Examples:
Condition   Self-catheteriza-
Home care   tion
Orthopedic   Activity program
appliances   Community
services

MENTAL DISABILITIES

See Developmental Problems/Needs.

Nursing Diagnoses

(Specify) Self-care Deficit related to sensory-
motor deficits

Impaired Communication related to impaired
receptive skills or impaired expressive skills

Potential Social Isolation (family, child) related
to fear and embarrassment of child's
behavior/appearance

Potential Altered Health Maintenance related to
insufficient knowledge of: (specify)

Examples:

Condition	Community
Child's potential	services
Home care	Education

MUSCULAR DYSTROPHY (Duchenne)

See also Developmental Problems/Needs.

Collaborative Problems

Potential Complications:

Seizures	*Metabolic failure*
Respiratory infections	

Nursing Diagnoses

Potential for Injury related to inability to control
movements

Potential Altered Nutrition: Less Than Body
Requirements related to sucking difficulties
(infant) and dysphagia

(Specify) Self-care Deficits related to sensory-
motor impairments

Impaired Verbal Communication related to
impaired ability to speak words secondary
to facial muscle involvement

Potential Impaired Physical Mobility related to
muscle weakness

Potential Altered Nutrition: More Than Body
Requirements related to increased caloric
consumption secondary to boredom in
presence of decreased metabolic needs
secondary to limited physical activity

Grieving (parental) related to progressive,
terminal nature of disease

Impaired Swallowing related to sensory-motor
deficits

Potential Hopelessness related to progressive
nature of disease

Potential Diversional Activity Deficit related to
effects of limitations on ability to participate
in recreational activities

Potential Altered Health Maintenance related to
insufficient knowledge of: (specify)

Examples:

Disease	Education
Pharmacological regimen	Community services
Activity program	

OBESITY

See also Developmental Problems/Needs.

Nursing Diagnoses

Ineffective Individual Coping related to increased
food consumption in response to stressors

Altered Health Maintenance related to the need
for

Exercise program	Behavioral modification
Nutrition counseling	

Self-concept Disturbance related to feelings of
self-degradation and response of others
(peers, family, others) to obesity

Altered Family Processes related to responses to
and effects of weight loss therapy on parent/
child relationship

Potential Impaired Social Interaction related to
inability to initiate and maintain
relationships secondary to feelings of
embarrassment and negative responses of
others

Potential Altered Health Maintenance related to
insufficient knowledge of: (specify)

Examples:
Condition
Etiology
Course
Risks
Therapies available

Destructive versus constructive eating
patterns
Self-help groups

OSTEOMYELITIS

See also Developmental Problems/Needs.

Collaborative Problems

Potential Complication: Infective emboli
Potential Complication: Side-effects of antibiotic
therapy (hematologic, renal, hepatic)

Nursing Diagnoses

Altered Comfort related to swelling,
hyperthermia, and infectious process of
bone
Diversional Activity Deficit related to impaired
mobility and long-term hospitalization
Potential Altered Nutrition: Less Than Body
Requirements related to anorexia secondary
to infectious process
Potential Colonic Constipation related to
immobility
Potential Impaired Skin Integrity related to
mechanical irritation of cast/splint
Potential for Injury: Pathological Fractures
related to disease process
Potential Altered Health Maintenance related to
insufficient knowledge of: (specify)
Examples:
Condition
Wound care
Activity
restrictions

Signs and
symptoms of
complications
Pharmacological
therapy
Follow-up care

PARASITIC DISORDERS

See also Developmental Problems/Needs.

Nursing Diagnoses

Potential Altered Nutrition: Less Than Body
Requirements related to anorexia, nausea,
vomiting, and deprivation of host nutrients
by parasites

Impaired Skin Integrity related to pruritus
secondary to emergence of parasites
(pinworms) onto perianal skin, lytic
necrosis, and tissue digestion

Diarrhea related to parasitic irritation to
intestinal mucosa

Altered Comfort: Abdominal Pain related to
parasitic invasion of small intestines

Potential for Infection Transmission related to
contagious nature of parasites

Potential Altered Health Maintenance related to
insufficient knowledge of: (specify)

Examples:
Condition
Mode of transmission
Prevention of reinfection
Hygiene
Clothing

POISONING

See also Dialysis, if indicated.
See also Unconscious Individual.

Collaborative Problems

Potential Complications:

Respiratory alkalosis   *Burns (acid/alkaline)*
Metabolic acidosis   *Aspiration*
Hemorrhage   *Blindness*
Fluid/electrolyte
imbalance

Nursing Diagnoses

Altered Comfort related to heat production
secondary to poisoning (*e.g.,* salicylate)

Potential for Injury related to

Examples:

Tonic/clonic movement	Bleeding tendencies

Fear related to invasive nature of treatments (gastric lavage, dialysis)

Anxiety (parental) related to uncertainty of situation and feelings of guilt

Potential for Injury related to lack of awareness of environmental hazards

Potential Altered Health Maintenance related to insufficient knowledge of: (specify)

Examples:
Condition
Treatments
Home treatment of accidental poisoning
Poison prevention
Storage
Teaching
Poisonous plants
Locks

RESPIRATORY TRACT INFECTION
(Lower)

See also Developmental Problems/Needs.
See also Adult Pneumonia.

Collaborative Problems

Potential Complications:

Hyperthermia	Septic shock
Respiratory insufficiency	Paralytic ileus

Nursing Diagnoses

Altered Comfort related to hyperthermia, malaise, and respiratory distress

Potential Altered Nutrition: Less Than Body Requirements related to anorexia secondary to dyspnea and malaise

Anxiety related to breathlessness and apprehension

Potential Fluid Volume Deficit related to insufficient intake secondary to dyspnea and malaise

Potential Altered Body Temperature related to
    infectious process
Potential Altered Health Maintenance related to
    insufficient knowledge of: (specify)
  Examples:
    Condition
    Prevention of recurrence
    Treatment
      Oxygen
      Croup tent

RHEUMATIC FEVER

See also Developmental Problems/Needs.

Collaborative Problems

Potential Complication: Endocarditis

Nursing Diagnoses

Diversional Activity Deficit related to prescribed
    bed rest
Altered Nutrition: Less Than Body
    Requirements related to anorexia
Altered Comfort related to arthralgia
Potential for Injury related to choreic
    movements
Potential Noncompliance: Long-term Antibiotic
    Therapy related to difficulty of maintaining
    preventive drug therapy when illness is
    resolved
Potential Altered Health Maintenance related to
    insufficient knowledge of: (specify)
  Examples:
    Condition
    Signs and symptoms of complications
    Long-term antibiotic therapy
    Prevention of recurrence
    Risk factors (surgery, *e.g.,* dental)

RHEUMATOID ARTHRITIS (Juvenile)

See also Developmental Problems/Needs.
See also Corticosteroid Therapy.

Collaborative Problems

Potential Complication: *Pericarditis*
Potential Complication: *Iridocyclitis*

Nursing Diagnoses

Impaired Physical Mobility related to pain and
restricted joint movement
Acute Pain related to swollen, inflamed joints
and restricted movement
Fatigue related to chronic inflammatory process
Potential Altered Health Maintenance related to
insufficient knowledge of: (specify)
Examples:

Condition	Rest versus
Pharmacological	activity
therapy	Myths
Exercise program	Community
	resources

REYE SYNDROME

See also Unconscious Individual, if indicated.

Collaborative Problems

Potential Complications:

Renal failure	Shock
Increased intracranial	Seizures
pressure	Coma
Fluid/electrolyte	Respiratory distress
imbalance	Diabetes insipidus
Hepatic failure	

Nursing Diagnoses

Anxiety (parental) related to diagnosis and
uncertain prognosis
Potential for Injury related to uncontrolled
tonic/clonic movements
Potential for Infection related to invasive
monitoring procedures
Altered Comfort related to hyperpyrexia and
malaise secondary to disease process
Fear related to separation from family, sensory

bombardment (ICU, treatments), and
unfamiliar experiences
Altered Family Process related to
Examples:
Critical nature of syndrome
Hospitalization of child
Separation of family members
Grieving related to actual, anticipated, or
possible death of child
Potential Impaired Skin Integrity related to
immobility
Potential Altered Health Maintenance related to
insufficient knowledge of: (specify)
Examples:
Condition
Etiology
Course
Treatments
Complications

SCOLIOSIS

See also Developmental Problems/Needs.

Nursing Diagnoses

Impaired Physical Mobility related to restricted
movement secondary to braces
Potential Impaired Skin Integrity related to
mechanical irritation of brace
Potential Noncompliance related to chronicity
and complexity of treatment regimen
Potential for Injury: Falls related to restricted
range of motion
Potential Altered Health Maintenance related to
insufficient knowledge of: (specify)
Examples:
Condition
Treatment
Medical
Surgical
Exercises
Environmental hazards
Care of appliances
Follow-up care
Community services

SICKLE CELL ANEMIA

See also Developmental Problems/Needs if the individual is a child.

Collaborative Problems

Potential Complications:

Sickling crisis
Transfusion therapy

Thrombosis and
  infarction
Cholelithiasis

Nursing Diagnoses

Altered Tissue Perfusion: Peripheral related to viscous blood and occlusion of microcirculation

Pain related to viscous blood and tissue hypoxia

(Specify) Self-care Deficit related to pain and immobility of exacerbations

Potential Altered Health Maintenance related to insufficient knowledge of: (specify)

  Examples:

    Hazards
    Signs and
      symptoms of
      complications

    Fluid require-
      ments
    Hereditary factors

TONSILLITIS

See also Tonsillectomy, if indicated.

Collaborative Problems

Potential Complication: Otitis media
Potential Complication: Rheumatic fever (β-hemolytic streptococci)*

Nursing Diagnoses

Acute Pain related to inflammation

Potential Fluid Volume Deficit related to inadequate fluid intake

Potential Altered Health Maintenance related to insufficient knowledge of: (specify)

Examples:
    Condition
    Treatments
        Medical
        Surgical
    Nutritional/fluid requirements
    Signs and symptoms of complications

WILMS' TUMOR

See also Developmental Problems/Needs.
See also Nephrectomy.
See also Cancer (General).

Collaborative Problems

Potential Complication: Metastases to liver, lung,
    bone, brain
Potential Complication: Sepsis

Nursing Diagnoses

Potential for Injury related to rupture of tumor
        capsule secondary to manipulation/
        palpation of abdomen
Anxiety (child) related to
    Examples:
        Age-related concerns
            Separation
            Strangers
            Pain
        Response of others to visible signs (alopecia)
        Uncertain future
Anxiety (parental) related to
    Examples:
        Unknown   Treatments
            prognosis   (chemotherapy)
        Painful   Feelings of
            procedures   inadequacy
Grieving related to actual, anticipated, or
        possible death of child
Spiritual Distress related to nature of disease and
        its possible disturbances on belief systems
Potential Altered Health Maintenance related to
        insufficient knowledge of: (specify)

Examples:

Condition	Nutritional
Prognosis	requirements
Treatments (side-	Follow-up care
effects)	Community
Home care	services

Psychiatric Disorders

AFFECTIVE DISORDERS (Depression)

Nursing Diagnoses

Grooming Self-care Deficit related to decreased interest in body, inability to make decisions, and feelings of worthlessness

Ineffective Individual Coping related to internal conflicts (guilt, low self-esteem) or feelings of rejection

Impaired Social Interactions related to alienation from others by constant complaining, rumination, or loss of pleasure from relationships

Ineffective Individual Coping: Excessive Physical Complaints (without organic etiology) related to inability to express emotional needs directly

Social Isolation related to inability to initiate activities to reduce isolation secondary to low energy levels

Dysfunctional Grieving related to unresolved grief, prolonged denial, and repression

Chronic Low Self-esteem related to feelings of worthlessness and failure

Ineffective Family Coping related to marital discord and role conflicts secondary to effects of chronic depression

Powerlessness related to unrealistic negative beliefs about self-worth or abilities

Altered Thought Processes related to negative

cognitive set (overgeneralizing, polarized thinking, selected abstraction, arbitrary inference)

Sexual Dysfunction related to decreased sex drive, loss of interest and pleasure

Diversional Activity Deficit related to a loss of interest or pleasure in usual activities and low energy levels

Impaired Home Maintenance Management related to inability to make decisions or concentrate

Potential for Self-harm related to feelings of hopelessness and loneliness

Sleep Pattern Disturbance related to difficulty in falling asleep or early morning awakening secondary to emotional stress

Colonic Constipation related to sedentary life-style, insufficient exercise, or inadequate diet

Potential Altered Nutrition: More Than Body Requirements related to increased intake versus decreased activity expenditures secondary to boredom and frustrations

Potential Altered Nutrition: Less Than Body Requirements related to anorexia secondary to emotional stress

Potential Altered Health Maintenance related to insufficient knowledge of: (specify)
  Examples:
    Condition
    Behavior modification
    Therapy options
      Pharmacological
      Electroshock
    Community resources

ANOREXIA NERVOSA

Collaborative Problems

Potential Complications:

Anemia   *Cardiac dysrhythmias*
Hypotension

Nursing Diagnoses

Altered Nutrition: Less Than Body
Requirements related to anorexia and self-
induced vomiting following eating and
laxative abuse

Self-concept Disturbance related to inaccurate
perception of self as obese

Potential Fluid Volume Deficit related to
vomiting and excessive weight loss

Sleep Pattern Disturbance related to fears and
anxiety concerning weight status

Activity Intolerance related to fatigue secondary
to malnutrition

Ineffective Individual Coping related to self-
induced vomiting, denial of hunger, and
insufficient food intake secondary to feelings
of loss of control and inaccurate perceptions
of body states

Ineffective Family Coping related to marital
discord and its effect on family members

Potential Impaired Skin Integrity related to dry
skin secondary to malnourished state

Colonic Constipation related to insufficient food
and fluid intake

Impaired Social Interactions related to inability
to form relationships with others or fear of
trusting relationships with others

Fear of Sexuality, Maturity related to
dissatisfaction with relationships with others
(parents, peers)

ANXIETY AND ADJUSTMENT DISORDERS

(Phobias, Anxiety States, Traumatic Stress
Disorders, Adjustment Reactions)

See also Substance Abuse Disorders, if indicated.

Nursing Diagnoses

Ineffective Individual Coping related to irrational
avoidance of objects or situations

Impaired Social Interactions related to effects of

behavior and actions on forming and
maintaining relationships

Ineffective Individual Coping related to
dependence on drugs

Anxiety related to irrational thoughts or guilt

Social Isolation related to irrational fear of social
situations

Ineffective Individual Coping related to
avoidance of objects or situations secondary
to a numbing of responsiveness following a
traumatic event

Sleep Pattern Disturbance related to recurrent
nightmares

Self-concept Disturbance related to feelings of
guilt

Ineffective Individual Coping related to altered
ability to constructively manage stressors
secondary to (specify)

Examples:

Physical illness	Natural disasters
Marital discord	Developmental
Business crisis	crisis

Potential Altered Health Maintenance related to
insufficient knowledge of: (specify)

Examples:

Condition

Pharmacological therapy

Legal system regarding violence

BIPOLAR DISORDER (Mania)

Nursing Diagnoses

Defensive Coping related to exaggerated sense of
self-importance and abilities secondary to
feelings of inadequacy and inferiority

Impaired Social Interaction related to overt
hostility, overconfidence, or manipulation
of others

Potential for Violence to Others related to
impaired reality testing, impaired judgment,
or inability to control behavior

Sleep Pattern Disturbance related to
hyperactivity

Altered Thought Processes related to flight of ideas, delusions, or hallucinations

Impaired Verbal Communication related to pressured speech

Potential Fluid Volume Deficit related to altered sodium excretion secondary to lithium therapy

Noncompliance related to feelings of no longer requiring medication

Potential Altered Health Maintenance related to insufficient knowledge of: (specify)
    Examples:
        Condition
        Pharmacological therapy

CHILDHOOD BEHAVIORAL DISORDERS
(Attention Deficit Disorders, Learning Disabilities)

Nursing Diagnoses

Altered Thought Processes related to inattention and impulsivity

Impaired Social Interactions related to inattention, impulsivity, or hyperactivity

Ineffective Individual Coping related to
    Examples:

Temper outbursts	Mood lability
Negativism	Stubbornness

Grieving (parental) related to anticipated losses secondary to condition

Altered Family Process related to adjustment requirements for situation
    Examples:

Time	Physical care
Energy	Prognosis
Money	

Potential for Violence related to impaired ability to control aggression

Potential Impaired Home Maintenance Management related to inadequate resources, inadequate, housing, or impaired caregivers

Potential Social Isolation (child, family) related
to disability and requirements for caregivers
Potential Altered Parenting: Abuse, Rejection, or
Overprotection related to inadequate
resources or inadequate coping mechanisms
Self-concept Disturbance related to effects of
limitations on achievement of
developmental tasks

OBSESSIVE-COMPULSIVE DISORDER

Nursing Diagnoses

(Specify) Self-care Deficit related to ritualistic
obsessions interfering with performance of
activities of daily living
Noncompliance related to poor concentration
and poor impulse control secondary to
obsessive thought patterns
Social Isolation related to fear of vulnerability
associated with need for closeness and
embarrassment over ritualistic behavior
Altered Thought Processes related to obsessive-
compulsive patterns as a conditioned relief-
seeking response to anxiety
Anxiety related to the perceived threat of actual
or anticipated events

PARANOID DISORDERS

Nursing Diagnoses

Impaired Social Interactions related to feelings of
mistrust and suspicions of others
Ineffective Denial related to inability to accept
own feelings and responsibility for actions
secondary to low self-esteem
Potential Altered Nutrition: Less Than Body
Requirements related to reluctance to eat
secondary to fear of poisoning
Altered Thought Processes related to inability to
evaluate reality secondary to feelings of
mistrust
Social Isolation related to fear and mistrust of
situations and others

PERSONALITY DISORDERS

Examples:

Schizoid	Histrionic
Antisocial	Passive-aggressive
Borderline	Paranoid
Narcissistic	Schizotypal
Avoidant	Dependent
Compulsive	

Nursing Diagnoses

Ineffective Individual Coping: Passive
  Dependence related to subordinating one's
  needs to decisions of others
Ineffective Individual Coping:
  Inappropriate intense anger
  Lack of impulse control
  Marked mood shifts
  Habitual disregard for social norms related to
    altered ability to meet responsibilities
    (role, social)
Impaired Social Interaction related to inability to
  maintain enduring attachments secondary
  to negative responses
Ineffective Individual Coping related to
  resistance (procrastination, stubbornness,
  intentional inefficiency) in responses to
  responsibilities (role, social)

SCHIZOPHRENIC DISORDERS

Nursing Diagnoses

Altered Thought Processes related to inability to
  evaluate reality
Potential for Violence to Others or Self-harm
  related to responding to delusional thoughts
  or hallucinations
Impaired Verbal Communication related to
  incoherent/illogical speech pattern, poverty
  of content of speech, and side-effects of
  medications
Impaired Social Interactions related to

Examples:

Withdrawal from external world	Inappropriate affect
Preoccupation with egocentric and illogical ideas	Inappropriate movements
	Extreme suspiciousness

Anxiety related to inability to cope with internal/external stressors

Impaired Home Maintenance Management related to impaired judgment, inability to self-initiate activity, and loss of skills over long course of illness

SOMATOFORM DISORDERS (Somatization, Hypochondriasis, Conversion Reactions)

See also Affective Disorders, if indicated.

Nursing Diagnoses

Impaired Social Interactions related to effects of multiple somatic complaints on relationships

Ineffective Individual Coping related to unrealistic fear of having a disease despite reassurance to contrary

Ineffective Individual Coping: Depression related to belief of not getting proper care or sufficient response from others for complaints

Ineffective Family Coping related to chronicity of illness

Noncompliance related to impaired judgments and thought disturbances

Dressing/Grooming Self-care Deficit related to loss of skills and lack of interest in body and appearance

Social Isolation related to withdrawal from environment

Diversional Activity Deficit related to apathy, inability to initiate goal-directed activities, and loss of skills

Self-concept Disturbance related to feelings of worthlessness and lack of ego boundaries

Potential Altered Health Maintenance related to insufficient knowledge of: (specify)

Examples:

Condition	Tardive
Pharmacological	dyskinesia
therapy	Occupational
	skills
	Social skills

SUBSTANCE ABUSE DISORDERS

Nursing Diagnoses

Altered Nutrition: Less Than Body Requirements related to anorexia

Potential Fluid Volume Deficit related to abnormal fluid loss secondary to vomiting and diarrhea

Potential for Injury related to disorientation, tremors, or impaired judgment

Potential for Self-harm related to disorientation, tremors, or impaired judgment

Potential for Violence related to

Examples:

Impulsive	Tremors
behavior	Impaired
Disorientation	judgment

Sleep Pattern Disturbances related to irritability, tremors, and nightmares

Anxiety related to loss of control

Ineffective Individual Coping: Anger, Dependence, or Denial related to inability to constructively manage stressors without drugs/alcohol

Sensory–Perceptual Alterations related to:

Examples:

Confusion	Impaired
Memory losses	judgments
	Overdose/
	withdrawal

Self-concept Disturbance related to guilt, mistrust, or ambivalence

Impaired Social Interactions related to
Examples:

Emotional	Impulsive
immaturity	behavior
Irritability	Aggressive
High anxiety	responses

Social Isolation related to loss of work or
withdrawal from others
Sexual Dysfunction related to impotence/loss of
libido secondary to altered self-concept and
substance abuse
Ineffective Family Coping related to disruption
in marital dyad and inconsistent limit
setting
Potential Altered Health Maintenance related to
insufficient knowledge of: (specify)
Examples:

Condition	High-risk
Treatments	situations
available	Community
	resources

Diagnostic and Therapeutic Procedures

ANGIOPLASTY (Percutaneous, Transluminal, Coronary, Peripheral)

Preprocedure Period

Nursing Diagnoses

Anxiety related to lack of knowledge of: (specify)
Examples:
Procedure
Preparation
Postprocedure care
Fear related to procedure, outcome, and possible
need for cardiac surgery

Postprocedure Period

Collaborative Problems

Potential Complications:

> *Dysrhythmias (coronary)*
> *Acute coronary occlusion (clot, spasm, collapse)*
> *Myocardial infarction (coronary)*
> *Arterial dissection or rupture*
> *Hemorrhage/hematoma (site)*
> *Paresthesia distal to site*
> *Arterial thrombosis*
> *Embolization (peripheral)*

Nursing Diagnoses

Impaired Physical Mobility related to prescribed immobility and restricted movement of involved extremity

Potential Altered Health Maintenance related to insufficient knowledge of: (specify)

Examples:

Condition	Medications
Home activities	Signs and
Diet	symptoms of
Site care	complications

ANTICOAGULANT THERAPY

Collaborative Problems

Potential Complication: Hemorrhage

Nursing Diagnoses

Potential Altered Health Maintenance related to insufficient knowledge of: (specify)

Examples:

Administration schedule
Identification medallion/card
Contraindications

Foods	Medications

Signs and symptoms of bleeding

Skin	Gastrointestinal
Neurological	

Potential hazards

Surgery	Pregnancy

ARTERIOGRAM

Preprocedure Period

Nursing Diagnoses

Anxiety related to lack of knowledge of: (specify)
Examples:
Procedure
Equipment
Possible sensations
Preparation
Post-care

Postprocedure Period

Collaborative Problems

Potential Complications:

Hematoma formation	*Urinary retention*
Hemorrhage	*Renal failure*
Stroke	*Paresthesia*
Thrombosis (arterial	*Embolism*
site)	*Allergic reaction*

Nursing Diagnoses

Potential Altered Health Maintenance related to insufficient knowledge of: (specify)
Examples:
Activity restrictions
Signs and symptoms of complications

CARDIAC CATHETERIZATION

Preprocedure Period

Nursing Diagnoses

Anxiety related to lack of knowledge of: (specify)
Examples:
Procedure
Purpose
Appearance of laboratory, positioning

Equipment
Length
Possible sensations
Preparation
NPO
Premedication
Postprocedure care (frequent vs activity
restriction)
Anxiety related to being awake during the
procedure

Postprocedure Period

Collaborative Problems

Potential Complications:

*Systemic (hypovolemia/hypervolemia, allergic
reaction)*
*Cardiac (dysrhythmias, myocardial infarction,
perforation)*
Cerebrovascular accident (CVA)
*Neurovascular (hematoma formation [site],
hemorrhage [site], paresis, or paresthesia)*

Nursing Diagnoses

Altered Comfort related to tissue trauma and
prescribed postprocedure immobilization
Potential Altered Health Maintenance related to
insufficient knowledge of: (specify)
Examples:
Site care
Signs and symptoms of complications
Follow-up care

CASTS

Collaborative Problems

Potential Complications:

Pressure (edema, mechanical)
Compartmental syndrome
Ulcer formation
Infection

Nursing Diagnoses

Potential for Injury related to hazards of crutch-walking and impaired mobility secondary to cast

Potential Impaired Skin Integrity related to pressure of cast on skin surface

Potential Impaired Home Maintenance Management related to the restrictions imposed by cast on performing activities of daily living and role responsibilities

(Specify) Self-care Deficits related to limitation of movement secondary to cast

Potential Altered Respiratory Function related to imposed immobility or restricted respiratory movement secondary to cast (body)

Diversional Activity Deficit related to boredom and inability to perform usual recreational activities

Potential Altered Health Maintenance related to insufficient knowledge of: (specify)

Examples:

Crutch-walking

Cast care

Exercise program

Signs and symptoms of complications

Numbness	Cyanosis
Tingling	Odor or pain
Burning	Inability to move
Blanching	distal parts

CHEMOTHERAPY

See also Cancer (General).

Collaborative Problems

Potential Complications:

Necrosis/phlebitis at intravenous site	*Peripheral nerve toxicosis*
Thrombocytopenia	*Anaphylaxis*
Anemia	*Pulmonary fibrosis*
Leukopenia	*Central nervous system toxicity*

Nursing Diagnoses

Potential Fluid Volume Deficit related to gastrointestinal fluid losses secondary to vomiting

Altered Nutrition: Less Than Body Requirements related to anorexia, nausea, and altered taste sensations

Potential for Infection related to altered immune system secondary to effects of cytotoxic agents or disease process

Potential Altered Family Processes related to interruptions imposed by treatment and schedule on patterns of living

Potential Sexual Dysfunction related to amenorrhea and sterility (temporary/permanent) secondary to effects of chemotherapy on testes/ovaries

Potential for Injury related to bleeding tendencies

Constipation/Diarrhea related to decreased bowel activity or irritation of epithelium of bowel

Altered Oral Mucous Membrane related to irritation of mucosa from medication

Fatigue related to anemia and chemical changes secondary to chemotherapy

CORTICOSTEROID THERAPY

Collaborative Problems

Potential Complications:

Peptic ulcer	Hypertension
Avascular necrosis	Thromboembolism
Diabetes mellitus	Hypokalemia
Osteoporosis	

Nursing Diagnoses

Potential Fluid Volume Excess: Edema related to sodium and water retention

Potential for Infection related to immunosuppression secondary to excessive adrenocortical hormones

Potential Altered Nutrition: More Than Body Requirements related to increased appetite

Situational Low Self-esteem related to appearance changes (*e.g.,* abnormal fat distribution, increased production of androgens)

Potential Altered Health Maintenance related to insufficient knowledge of: (specify)
Examples:
Administration schedule
Indications for therapy
Side-effects
Signs and symptoms of complications
Hazards of adrenal insufficiency
Potential causes of adrenal insufficiency

Injuries	Abrupt cessation
Surgery	of therapy
Vomiting	

Emergency kit
Dietary requirements
Prevention of infection

ELECTROCONVULSIVE THERAPY (ECT)

Preprocedure Period

Nursing Diagnoses

Potential Noncompliance related to preprocedure food/fluid restrictions secondary to memory deficits and confusion

Anxiety related to anticipated treatment and unknown prognosis

Anxiety related to lack of knowledge of: (specify)
Examples:
Preprocedure/postprocedure
Sensations expected
Food, fluid restrictions

Postprocedure Period

Collaborative Problems

Potential Complication: Hypertension
Potential Complication: Dysrhythmias

Nursing Diagnoses

Potential for Injury related to uncontrolled tonic/clonic movements and disorientation, confusion posttreatment

Altered Comfort: Headaches, Muscle Aches, Nausea related to seizure activity and Tissue Trauma secondary to electrical current

Potential for Aspiration related to post-ECT somnolence

Altered Thought Processes related to memory losses and disorientation secondary to effects of ECT on cerebral function

ELECTRONIC FETAL MONITORING
(Internal)

See also Intrapartum Period (General).

Preinsertion
Nursing Diagnoses

Anxiety related to need for internal electronic fetal monitoring and lack of information

Postinsertion
Collaborative Problems

Potential Complication: Fetal scalp laceration
Potential Complication: Perforated uterus

Nursing Diagnoses

Impaired Physical Mobility related to restrictions secondary to monitor cords

ENTERAL NUTRITION
Collaborative Problems

Potential Complications:

Hypoglycemia/hyperglycemia
Hypervolemia
Hypertonic dehydration
Electrolyte and trace mineral imbalances
Mucosal erosion

Nursing Diagnoses

Potential for Infection related to gastrostomy incision and enzymatic action of gastric juices on skin

Altered Comfort: Cramping, Distention, Nausea, Vomiting related to type of formula, rate, or temperature

Diarrhea related to adverse response to formula, rate, or temperature

Potential for Aspiration related to position of tube and of individual

Altered Comfort related to incision and tension on gastrostomy tube

Potential Self-concept Disturbance related to inability to taste or swallow food/fluids

Potential Altered Health Maintenance related to insufficient knowledge of: (specify)

Examples:
Nutritional indications/requirements
Home care
Signs and symptoms of complications
Infection
Diarrhea
Mechanical problems

HEMODIALYSIS

See also Chronic Renal Failure.

Collaborative Problems

Potential Complications (During/After Treatment):

Fluid imbalances (disequilibrium syndrome)
Electrolyte imbalance (potassium, sodium)
Nausea/vomiting
Transfusion reaction
Aneurysm
Hemorrhage
Vascular access (fistulas, graft, shunts, venous catheters)
Bleeding
Dialysate leakage
Clots
Disconnection
Infection
Hepatitis B
Fever/chills

Nursing Diagnoses

Potential for Injury to (Vascular) Access Site
related to vulnerability

Potential for Infection related to direct access to
bloodstream secondary to vascular access

Powerlessness related to need for treatments to
live despite effects on life-style

Altered Family Processes related to the
interruptions of treatment schedule on role
responsibilities

Potential Altered Health Maintenance related to
insufficient knowledge of: (specify)

Examples:

Rationale of treatment

Access site
Care (general, posttreatment)
Precautions
Emergency treatments (disconnected,
bleeding, clotting)

Pretreatment instructions
Diet   Medications

Assessments
Bruit   Weights
Blood pressure

HEMODYNAMIC MONITORING

See also Medical Diagnosis of the individual.

Collaborative Problems

Potential Complications:

Sepsis
Hemorrhage (site)
Emboli
Thrombosis (clotting)
Bleeding back
Vasospasm
Tissue ischemia/hypoxia
*System problems (leaks, air bubbles,
misconnection, damaged/unbalanced
transducer, damaged amplifier, damaged
stopcock, flush device, or pressure tubing)*

Nursing Diagnoses

Potential for Infection related to direct access to bloodstream

Impaired Physical Mobility related to position restrictions during monitoring

Potential Altered Health Maintenance related to insufficient knowledge of: (specify)
Examples:
Purpose
Procedure
Associated care

HICKMAN CATHETER

Collaborative Problems

Potential Complication: *Air embolism*
Potential Complication: *Nonpatent catheter*

Nursing Diagnoses

Potential for Infection related to direct access to bloodstream

Potential Impaired Home Maintenance Management related to lack of knowledge of catheter management

INTRA-AORTIC BALLOON PUMPING

Preprocedure Period

Nursing Diagnoses

Anxiety related to lack of knowledge of: (specify)
Examples:
Procedure (preparation)
Nursing care

Intraprocedure/Postprocedure Period

Collaborative Problems

Potential Complications:

Death
Arterial insufficiency/ thrombosis

Emboli
Gastrointestinal bleeding

Sepsis/infection
Peripheral neuropathy/
  claudication
Thrombocytopenia
Bleeding

Disseminated
  intravascular
  coagulation
Mechanical
  malfunction
Dysrhythmias

Nursing Diagnoses

Impaired Physical Mobility related to prescribed
  immobility and restricted movement of
  involved extremity

Potential for Infection related to direct access to
  bloodstream

Potential Colonic Constipation related to
  immobility and restricted movement of
  involved limb

Potential Sensory–Perceptual Alteration related
  to
  Examples:
    Immobility   Disruption of
    Pain   biorhythms
    Excessive
      environmental
      stimuli

Fear related to treatments, environment, and
  risk of death

Altered Family Processes related to the critical
  nature of situation and uncertain prognosis

MECHANICAL VENTILATION

See also Tracheostomy.

Collaborative Problems

Potential Complications:

Acidosis/alkalosis
Disconnected
  ventilator
Airway obstruction/
  atelectasis
Tracheal necrosis

Infection
Gastrointestinal
  bleeding
Tension pneumothorax
Oxygen toxicity
Respirator dependency

Nursing Diagnoses

Impaired Verbal Communication related to
inability to speak secondary to intubation

Potential Impaired Skin Integrity related to
imposed immobility

Potential for Infection related to disruption of
skin layer secondary to tracheostomy

Altered Family Processes related to critical
nature of situation and uncertain prognosis

Anxiety/Fear related to condition, treatments,
environment, and risk of death

Potential Sensory–Perceptual Alterations related
to excessive environmental stimuli and
decreased input of meaningful stimuli
secondary to treatment and critical care unit

Powerlessness related to respirator dependency

PACEMAKER INSERTION

Preprocedure Period

Nursing Diagnoses

Fear related to impending pacemaker insertion
and prognosis

Postprocedure Period

Collaborative Problems

Potential Complications:

Cardiac (perforation, dysrhythmias)
*Pacemaker (failure, electromagnetic interference,
undersensing/oversensing, partial/improper
sensing or wire break)*
Rejection of unit
Pressure necrosis of skin over unit
Site (hemorrhage)

Nursing Diagnoses

Altered Comfort related to pain at insertion site
and prescribed postprocedure
immobilization

Self-concept Disturbance related to perceived
loss of health and dependence on
pacemaker

Impaired Physical Mobility related to incisional
site pain, activity restrictions, and fear of
lead displacements

Potential for Infection related to operative site

Potential Altered Health Maintenance related to
insufficient knowledge of: (specify)

Examples:

Site care

Signs and symptoms of skin complications

Electromagnetic interference

Microwave ovens	Electric motors
	Antitheft devices
Arc welding equipment	Power transmitters
Gasoline engines	

Pacemaker function

Daily pulse taking

Signs of impending battery failure

Activity restrictions

Follow-up care

PERITONEAL DIALYSIS

Collaborative Problems

Potential Complications:

Fluid imbalances
Electrolyte imbalances
Hemorrhage
Negative nitrogen balance
*Inflow/outflow problems (displacement, plugging,
 fibrin clots)*
Bowel/bladder perforation
Hyperglycemia
Peritonitis

Nursing Diagnoses

Potential for Infection related to direct access to
peritoneal cavity, need to disconnect
catheter for treatment, and growth medium

potential of the dialysate (high glucose
concentration)

Potential for Injury to catheter site related to
vulnerability

Potential Impaired Breathing Patterns related to
immobility and pressure on diaphragm
during dwell time

Altered Comfort related to
Examples:
Rapid instillation
Pressure from fluid
Excessive suction during outflow
Extreme temperature of solution (hot or
cold)

Potential Altered Nutrition: Less Than Body
Requirements related to anorexia secondary
to abdominal distention during dialysis,
protein loss in dialysate, or vomiting

Potential Fluid Volume Excess related to fluid
retention secondary to catheter problems
(kinks, blockages) and/or position

Altered Family Processes related to interruptions
of treatment schedule on role
responsibilities

Powerlessness related to need for treatment to
live despite effects on life-style

Impaired Home Maintenance Management
related to lack of knowledge of treatment
procedure

Potential Altered Health Maintenance related to
insufficient knowledge of: (specify)
Examples:
Rationale of treatment
Home care
Self-care activities
Protection of catheter
Aseptic technique
Activity needs
Prescribed diet
Control of fluid intake/output
Medication regimen
Signs/symptoms of complications
Follow-up visits
Daily recording
Intake

Output
Blood pressure
Weights

RADIATION THERAPY (External)

Preprocedure Period

Nursing Diagnoses

Anxiety related to lack of knowledge of: (specify)
Examples:
Procedure
Site-related, local/systemic effects of therapy
(skin, gastrointestinal, neurological,
oral membranes)

Post–procedure Period

Collaborative Problems

*Potential Complication of Head/Brain Irradiation:
Increased intracranial pressure*

Nursing Diagnoses

Potential Impaired Skin Integrity related to
radiation exposure
Self-concept Disturbance related to alopecia
secondary to irradiation to head and visible
markings outlining treatment field
Altered Oral Mucous Membrane related to
mucositis, gingivitis, esophagitis, and dry
mouth secondary to irradiation (head/neck,
chest/back)
Fatigue related to tissue damage, hypoxia
secondary to radiation
Nausea and Vomiting related to irradiation of
abdomen/lower back
Diarrhea related to increased peristalsis
secondary to irradiation of abdomen/lower
back
Potential for Infection related to moist skin
reaction
Potential Altered Nutrition: Less Than Body
Requirements related to anorexia, nausea/
vomiting, or stomatitis

Activity Intolerance related to fatigue secondary
    to treatments or transportation
Potential Altered Health Maintenance related to
    insufficient knowledge of: (specify)
    Examples:
        Skin care
        Signs of complications

TRACHEOSTOMY

Preoperative Period

Nursing Diagnoses

Anxiety related to lack of knowledge of
    impending surgery and implications of
    condition on life-style (chronic)

Postoperative Period

Collaborative Problems

Potential Complications:

Hypoxia
Hemorrhage
Tracheal edema

Nursing Diagnoses

Potential Ineffective Airway Clearance related to
    increased secretions secondary to
    tracheostomy, obstruction of inner cannula,
    or displacement of tracheostomy tube
Potential for Infection related to excessive
    pooling of secretions and bypassing of upper
    respiratory defenses
Impaired Verbal Communications related to
    inability to produce speech secondary to
    tracheostomy
Potential Altered Sexuality Patterns related to
    change in appearance, fear of rejection
Potential Altered Health Maintenance related to
    insufficient knowledge of: (specify)
    Examples:
        Tracheostomy care
        Signs and symptoms of complication

TRACTION

See also Fractures.

Collaborative Problems

Potential Complications:

Thrombophlebitis
Renal calculi
Urinary tract infection
Neurovascular compromise

Nursing Diagnoses

Potential Impaired Skin Integrity related to
imposed immobility
Potential for Infection related to susceptibility to
microorganism secondary to skeletal
traction pins
Potential Colonic Constipation related to
decreased peristalsis secondary to
immobility and analgesics
Potential Altered Respiratory Function related to
imposed immobility and pooling of
respiratory secretions

TOTAL PARENTERAL NUTRITION
(Hyperalimentation Therapy)

Collaborative Problems

Potential Complications:

Sepsis
Hypoglycemia/
  hyperglycemia
Air embolism
Osmotic diuresis

Perforation
Pneumothorax,
  hydrothorax,
  hemothorax

Nursing Diagnoses

Potential for Infection related to catheter's direct
access to bloodstream
Potential Impaired Skin Integrity related to
continuous skin surface irritation secondary
to catheter and adhesive

Potential Self-concept Disturbance related to
inability to ingest food
Potential Altered Oral Mucous Membrane
related to inability to ingest food/fluid
Potential Altered Health Maintenance related to
insufficient knowledge of: (specify)
Examples:
Home care
Signs and symptoms of complications
Catheter care
Follow-up care (laboratory studies)

Appendix

Adult Data-base Assessment Guide

This guide directs the nurse to collect data to assess functional health patterns* of the individual and to determine the presence of actual, potential, or possible nursing diagnoses. When the person has a medical problem, the nurse will also have to assess for data in order to collaborate with the physician in monitoring the problem.

As with any printed assessment tool, the nurse must determine whether to collect or defer collecting certain data. The symbol △ identifies data that should be collected on hospitalized persons. The collection of data in sections not marked with △ should probably be deferred with most acutely ill persons or when the information is irrelevant to the individual.

As the nurse interviews the person, significant data may surface. The nurse should then ask other questions (focus assessment) to determine the presence of a pattern. For further information, the reader is referred to Section II of *Nursing Diagnosis: Application to Clinical Practice,* 3rd ed., by Lynda Juall Carpenito (Philadelphia, JB Lippincott, 1989).

For example, the client reports during the initial interview that she has a problem with incontinence. The nurse should then ask specific questions utilizing the focus assessment for Altered Patterns of Urinary Elimination to determine which diagnosis of incontinence is present. After the nurse has identified the factors, the plan of care can be initiated.

* The functional health patterns have been adapted from Gordon M: Nursing Diagnosis: Application and Process. New York, McGraw-Hill, 1982.

Data-base Assessment Format

1. **Health Perception–Health Management Pattern**

   A. Health management

   "How would you usually describe your health?"

Excellent	Fair
Good	Poor

   "How would you describe your health at this time?"

   Review the daily health practices of the individual (adults, children).

Dental care	Exercise regimen
Food intake	Leisure activities
Fluid intake	Responsibility in the family

   Use of

Tobacco	Alcohol
Salt, sugar, fat products	Drugs (over-the-counter, prescribed)

   Knowledge of safety practices

Fire prevention	Automobile (maintenance, seatbelts)
Water safety	
Children	Bicycle
	Poison control

   Knowledge of disease and preventive behavior

   Specific diseases (*e.g.,* heart disease, cancer, respiratory disease, childhood diseases, infections, dental disease)

   Susceptibility (*e.g.,* presence of risk factors, family history)

   "What do you do to keep healthy and to prevent disorders in yourself? In your children?"

Adequate nutrition	Professional examinations (gynecological, dental)
Weight control	
Exercise program	Immunizations
Self-examinations (breasts, testicles)	

B. Developmental history*
Family history (diagrammatic outline of
family structure, indicating illnesses of
living; deceased; cause and age)

Maternal	Paternal
grandparents	grandparents
Mother	Father
Spouse	Siblings

Patient
Children
Assess for achievement of developmental
tasks.

Young adult
(Intimacy vs. isolation)
Accepting self and stabilizing self-concept
Establishing independence from parental
home and financial aid
Becoming established in a vocation or
profession that provides personal
satisfaction, economic independence,
and a feeling of making a worthwhile
contribution to society
Learning to appraise and express love,
responsibility through more than
sexual contexts
Establishing an intimate bond with
another, either through marriage or
with a close friend
Establishing and managing a residence,
home
Finding a congenial social group
Deciding whether to have children
Formulating a meaningful philosophy of
life
Becoming involved as a citizen in the
community

Middle age
(Generativity vs stagnation)
Developing a sense of unity and abiding
intimacy with mate

* From Nursing History Guide, Nursing Department,
Southeastern Missouri University, Cape Giraudeau, Missouri

Helping growing and grown children become happy and responsible adults—relinquishing central position in their life

Taking pride in accomplishments of self and spouse

Finding pleasure in generativity and recognition in work

Balancing work with other roles

Preparing for retirement

Role reversal with parents—parental loss

Achieving mature social and civic responsibility

Developing or maintaining active organizational membership

Accepting and adjusting to changes of middle age (physical)

Socialization with new and old friends

Use of leisure time

Older adult

(Integrity vs despair)

Deciding how and where to live out remaining years

Continuing supportive, close, and warm relationships with significant others including a satisfying sexual relationship, if desired

Satisfactory living arrangements—safe, comfortable household routine

Supplemental retirement income if possible

Maintaining maximal level of self-health care

Maintaining interest in people outside of family

Maintaining social, civic, and political responsibility

Pursuing interests

Finding meaning in life after retirement

Facing inevitable illness and death of self and significant others

Formulating a philosophy of life

Finding meaning to life through philosophy/religion

Adjusting to death of spouse or other
loved one
C. Health perception
△ Reason for and expectations of
hospitalization (and previous hospital
experiences)
△ "Describe your illness."
Cause   Onset
△ "What treatments or practices have been
prescribed?"
Diet   Surgery
Weight   Cessation of
loss   smoking
Medications   Exercises
△ "Have you been able to follow the
prescribed instructions?" If not,
"What has prevented you?"
△ "Have you experienced or do you
anticipate a problem with caring for
yourself (your children, your home)?"
Mobility   Financial
problems   concerns
Sensory   Structural
deficits   barriers
(vision,   (stairs,
hearing)   narrow
doorways)
△ "Are there any problems that could
contribute to falls or accidents?"
Unfamiliar setting
Decreased sensorium (vertigo,
confusion)
Sensory deficits (visual, auditory,
tactile)
Motor deficits (gait, tremors, range
of motion, coordination)
Urinary/bowel urgency
2. △ **Nutritional–Metabolic Pattern**
"What is the usual daily food intake (meals,
snacks)?"
"What is the usual fluid intake (type,
amounts)?"
"How is your appetite?"
Indigestion   Vomiting
Nausea   Sore mouth

"What are your food restrictions or
preferences?"
"Any supplements (vitamins, feedings)?"
"Has your weight changed in the past 6
months?" If yes, "Why? How much?"
"Any problems with ability to eat?"

Swallow liquids	Chew
Swallow solids	Feed self

Skin

"What is the skin condition?"

Color,	Edema (type,
temperature,	location)
turgor	Pruritus (location)
Lesions (type,	
description,	
location)	

△ "Are there any factors present that could
contribute to pressure ulcer
development?"

Immobility	Dehydration
Malnourished	Decreased
Sensory deficits	circulation

3. △ **Elimination Pattern**

Bladder

"Are there any problems or complaints
with the usual pattern of urinating?"

Oliguria	Retention
Polyuria	Burning
Dysuria	Incontinence
Dribbling	

"Do you use assistive devices?"

Intermittent	Incontinence
catheterization	briefs
Catheter (Foley,	Cystostomy
external)	

Bowel

"What is the usual time, frequency, color,
consistency, pattern?"
"Assistive devices (type, frequency)?"

Ileostomy	Cathartics
Colostomy	Laxatives
Enemas	Suppositories

4. **Activity–Exercise Pattern**

"Describe usual daily/weekly activities of daily living."

Occupation	Exercise pattern
Leisure activities	(type, frequency)

△ "Are there any limitations in ability?"

Ambulating (gait, weight-bearing, balance)

Bathing self (shower, tub)

Dressing/grooming (oral hygiene)

Toileting (commode, toilet, bedpan)

"Are there complaints of dyspnea or fatigue?"

△ "Are there factors present that could interfere with self-care after discharge?"

Motor deficits	Cognitive/sensory deficits
Emotional deficits	
Lack of knowledge	Environmental barriers
	Lack of resources

5. △ **Sleep–Rest Pattern**

"What is the usual sleep pattern?"

Bedtime	Sleep aids
Hours slept	(medication, food)
	Sleep routine

"Any problems?"

Difficulty falling asleep	Not feeling rested after sleep
Difficulty remaining asleep	

6. △ **Cognitive–Perceptual Pattern**

"Any deficits in sensory perception (hearing, sight, touch)?"

Glasses	Hearing aid

"Any complaints?"

Vertigo	Insensitivity to cold or heat
Insensitivity to superficial pain	

"Able to read and write?"

7. **Self-perception Pattern**

△ "What are you most concerned about?"

"What are your present health goals?"

△ "How would you describe yourself?"

"Has being ill made you feel different about yourself?"

"To what do you attribute the following?"

Becoming ill	Maintaining
Getting better	health

8. Role–Relationship Pattern

△ Communication

"Any hearing deficits?" (aids, lip-reads)

"What language do you speak?"

"Is speech clear? Relevant?"

Assess ability to express self and understand others (orally, in writing, with gestures)

Relationships

"Do you live alone?" If not, "With whom?"

"Whom do you turn to for help in time of need?"

Assess family life (members, educational level, occupations)

Cultural background	Decision-making
Activities (lone or group)	Communication patterns
Role discipline	Finances

"Any complaints?"

Parenting difficulties	Marital difficulties
Difficulties with relatives (in-laws, parents)	Abuse (physical, verbal, substance)

9. Sexuality–Sexual Functioning

"Has there been or do you anticipate a change in your sexual relations because of your condition?"

Fertility	Pregnancy
Libido	Contraceptives
Erections	
Menstruation	

Assess knowledge of sexual functioning

10. Coping–Stress Management Pattern

△ "How do you make decisions (alone, with assistance, with whom)?"

△ "Has there been a loss in your life in the

past year (or changes—moves, job, health)?"

"What do you like about yourself?"

"What would you like to change in your life?"

"What is preventing you?"

"What do you do when you are tense or under stress (e.g., problem-solve, eat, sleep, take medication, seek help)?"

△ "What can the nurses do to provide you with more comfort and security during your hospitalization?"

11. Value–Belief System

"With what (whom) do you find a source of strength or meaning?"

"Is religion or God important to you?"

"What are your religious practices (type, frequency)?"

"Have your values or moral beliefs been challenged recently? Describe."

△ "Is there a religious person or practice (diet, book, ritual) that you would desire during hospitalization (institutionalization)?"

12. △ Physical Assessment (Objective)

General appearance

Weight and height

Eyes (appearance, drainage)

  Pupils (size: equal; reactive to light)

  Vision (glasses)

Mouth

  Mucous membrane (color, moisture, lesions)

  Teeth (condition: loose, broken; dentures)

Hearing (hearing aids)

Pulses (radial, apical, peripheral)

  Rate, rhythm, volume

Respirations

  Rate, quality, breath sounds (upper and lower lobes)

Blood pressure

Temperature

Bowel sounds

Skin (color, temperature, turgor)

  Lesions, edema, pruritus

Functional ability (mobility and safety)
  Dominant hand
  Use of right and left hands, arms, legs
  Strength, grasp
  Range of motion
  Gait (stability)
  Use of aids (wheelchair, braces, cane,
      walker)
  Weight-bearing (full, partial, none)
Mental status
  Orientation (time, place, person, events)
  Memory
  Affect
  Eye contact

Index

Nursing diagnostic categories appear in **boldface**.

Index

Index

Index

Index